THE NO NONSENSE GUIDE TO HEALTHY LIVING

A COMPLETE GUIDE FOR CREATING A HEALTHY LIFE FOR YOU AND YOUR FAMILY

MARLENE MACMILLAN
WITH
BILL TARA

Illustrations by Neil Fraser
and Keri Struth
Book Cover design by Katie Gaughan
at 999 Design

The Academy of Wellness

This book is published by
Grosvenor House Publishing Ltd
28 – 30 High Street, Guildford, Surrey, GU1 3HY.
www.grosvenorhousepublishing.co.uk

A CIP record for this book
Is available from the British Library

ISBN 978-1-905529-15-5

About the Authors

Marlene Macmillan

Marlene, Personal Trainer to Scotland's movers and shakers, a teacher of the Chi Ball Method, which is an holistic approach to exercise using Tai Chi, Yoga, Pilates and Deep Relaxation, is a great believer in Chinese Medicine and the philosophy of Energy Medicine; an advocate of the macrobiotic diet favoured by the likes of Madonna and Gwyneth Paltrow, she swears that by living with the rhythm of nature, health and happiness can be established.

Her passion for health was intensified following a series of serious health problems and a personal bout of depression. Learning to live again led her deeper into her long time interest in health and healing.

Marlene has been teaching for over two decades and has taught in the UK, Australia and the USA. Her burning desire is to put Scotland on the map as the nation leading the way in educating people about the importance of nutrition and hydration. Her background, apart from teaching Lifestyle Workshops, is in Sales and Marketing. She worked with the *Herald* newspaper before building a successful business with Reebok, the sportswear giants in the late eighties and early nineties. Her favourite saying is, "If you don't look after your body, then where are you going to live?"

Bill Tara

Bill Tara is a pioneer in natural health care. He has worked as an entrepreneur, educator, author and health counsellor. In the mid 1960s he was a founder and Vice President of Erewhon Natural Foods, one of the first American distributors of organic food products. He was closely involved with the development of manufacturing and retailing of natural food products in both North America and Europe.

In the mid 1970s he became a leader in the worldwide macrobiotic movement. He has served as Chairman of the European Macrobiotic Assembly and the North American Macrobiotic Congress as well as Chairman of the Macrobiotic Teachers Certification Board. He has represented natural health care through testimony before the American Congress, in the media (including an appearance on ABC television's *Nightline* with Ted Koppel) and as a speaker at numerous conferences on health and the environment worldwide.

He is co-founder of the Kushi Institute and the creator of the Community Health Foundation in London, England, where he served as Executive Director for six years. He has taught seminars in over twenty countries and been on the faculty of Naropa University in Boulder, Colorado, and the International Macrobiotic Institute in Kiental, Switzerland. His writing credits include *Your Face Never Lies* and *Macrobiotics and Human Behaviour*.

ILLUSTRATIONS

Neil Fraser & Keri Struth are a, soon – to - be, husband and wife team. Neil is a teacher by day and a crime fighting superhero by night (otherwise known as the illustrator). Both Keri and Neil honed their skills through a number of methods. Keri took an MSc at Salford and a BAhons at Glasgow School of Art and Neil took a BAhons at Dundee University. Equal in influence was a misspent youth influenced by reading comics and developing their own style.

The Academy of Wellness Corporate and Personal Services

Corporate Wellness Programmes

Enlightened management realizes the importance of creating a workplace that promotes health and reduces stress. British industry loses more than £4 billion a year due to sickness. Health is a "bottom line" as well as a humanitarian issue.

The Academy of Wellness offers a variety of services designed to promote a healthier and stress-free workplace. Our programmes focus on simple commonsense approaches to wellbeing that educate, empower and inspire individuals to create a more healthy way of living. We can tailor-make programmes to fit the specific needs of you and your company, from in-house workshops to corporate awaydays.

Optimal Health Seminars

The Academy of Wellness can provide your church, social club or educational group with lectures or seminars on a wide variety of topics dealing with alternative health care, family health issues and a variety of timely topics. Both Marlene and Bill are experienced public presenters and give lively and informative presentations.

Personal or Family Health Consultations

We can provide individual and family health consultations by appointment with either Bill or Marlene. These sessions are designed to discuss positive and practical health strategies for dealing with either specific or general health concerns.

Personal Training Sessions

Marlene is an experienced personal trainer and teacher of a variety of physical disciplines that can help in weight loss, increased vitality and stamina. Each session ends with stress reduction, rest and relaxation techniques. These sessions are by appointment only and include an introductory consultation and health assessment.

Health Coaching

Starting in 2006 the Academy of Wellness will provide follow-up health coaching for our clients with fortnightly telephone conferences. These conference calls will provide an easy way to have questions answered, get personal coaching and be exposed to the newest information that we have put together. (The coaching programme begins in April 2006.)

Continuing Professional Development

Health and Education professionals have to continue their CPD requirements. We can provide programmes that will specifically meet the needs. Contact us for details on group programmes.

The Academy of Wellness
www.wellnessconsultant.co.uk.
or email malmac1@btopenworld.com

Acknowledgements

One of the biggest blessings of writing this book is the opportunity to say thank you to the people I have worked with, learned from and who have helped me "know what I know".

To my friend Julie Hanson, for taking me along to a workshop with Nick Williams when I was "lost" and got my life moving again – thanks Jools. To my friend Janis Sue Smith, thank you for introducing me to the wonderful Margaret Doherty, who opened my eyes to the amazing world of magnetic energy which set me on the road to recovery. To my oldest and dearest friend Anne Sneddon for her love, friendship and heartfelt support in all I have done; thanks, Snedds. To each and every one of my clients over many years who trusted me and allowed me to share in their life the many things that were holding them back from living a life of good health with an abundance of energy and happiness.

Thank you to my family who have listened to me for years rambling on with passion about my work and who now share this so powerfully with all and sundry. To my late dad, who inspired me always by telling me to believe that we can all achieve anything we put our minds to. To Mum, who will be 80 this year and who never once said to me, "It's too late to change," and now uses magnets, drinks clean living water, sleeps on a magnetic bed, walks everywhere and has a renewed spring in her step. To my brother Jacky who now has a pain-free back and no more stomach ache, thank you for listening to your wee sister. To my sister Shirley who has been an absolute follower and believer in my work from day one and whose passionate belief in my work and my book has inspired me and encouraged me, thank you. To my sister Sandie who, after many years, has seen the light and that makes me smile; she has now become my number one fan, thank you. To my sister Lainey, who spreads the word all over the world and carries my brochures with her on her travels and who has converted many of her colleagues to my no-nonsense approach to health, thank you. To my sister Marguerite, whom I still have to "capture" and I will, you will be in the gang soon, big sis, thank you. To my late sister Margo, thank you for the amazing creative talent you instilled in your daughter Keri that enabled her with her fiancé Neil to bring these wonderful cartoon characters for my book to life.

To my partner Bill Tara I owe a mega thank you for his huge contribution as editor and for his continued sense of humour as he read through my work. He lets me do what I do best: talk! I write with increased excitement as my ideas appear on screen. Without Bill's editing, my book would have been the size of the *Encyclopaedia Britannica*, and that was only the chapter on why we should drink water!

To all my many friends, home and afar, Vicki in Sydney and Peter in Perth, they really are an extraordinary bunch, and I feel very blessed to have you all in my life, thank you for your love, support and belief in me.

I'd also like to acknowledge and say thank you to all the companies I have worked with delivering Corporate Programmes on health and well being for their staff.

FOREWORD

When Marlene asked me to help her putting her book together I was more than happy. For the past forty years I have been involved in the wellness revolution in one way or another. What I have come to believe is that the problems of creating a healthy society do not hinge on some new scientific discovery.

The causes of the epidemic of degenerative disease in Europe and North America are well known – the solutions are at hand. Just imagine what a benefit to everyone if heart disease, cancer and diabetes were reduced by 50%. Think of the grief spared, the lives saved and the money used for more pressing matters. It is possible to do it with enlightened government, committed health workers and most importantly a critical mass of the population who are willing to take action. The catalyst for all this is having the message communicated in a way that hits home with the general public.

Over the past thirty years, with all the developments and improvement in the treatment of disease there has been little movement toward prevention. Dedicated non-professionals like Marlene have generated the greatest strides toward a healthy society. Grassroots movements have promoted the push toward better nutrition, the importance of exercise, the mind/body connection and low impact alternative treatment and the anti-smoking movement. It was only later that orthodox medicine came around. The sad truth is that all of the above were dismissed as not based on science or as being insignificant. Thank goodness no one gave up.

What makes Marlene different from so many of the health gurus out there is that she has not lost her sense of humour or compassion. She has experienced sickness and depression and come out the other side with her huge gratitude for life still intact. She is not bogged down with some overriding "theory" to prove. For her there is no dogma. She teaches what she does and has an open mind. When she teaches, the most common sound in the room is laughter, from her and her students. Her desire to help others is as genuine as her no-nonsense approach to what works.

You will enjoy this book. The information is simple, direct and effective. If you follow Marlene's advice you will be better for it. After all, that's what she guarantees.

Bill Tara

CONTENTS

CHAPTER ONE

WHY WRITE A BOOK?

Five years ago I experienced a single moment that changed my life. I was walking in the woods with my two beautiful dogs. There was a winter chill in the air and I was deep in a depression that had lead me into a spiritual and physical black hole. My body had only partially recovered from a series of accidents and surgeries and my mind and spirit were still reeling from a year of emotional devastation.

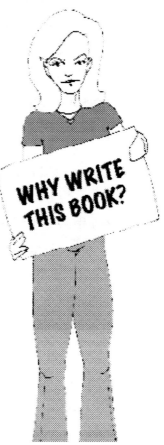

Across the field a herd of deer emerged from the woods and Molly and Tess leapt forward on the chase. The dogs were too old and deer too quick, springing out of sight in an instant. They came back to me filled with joy at their adventure, tails wagging and eyes alert. I could still see the deer in the distance already grazing. They were beautiful in the afternoon light – healthy and strong.

The woods were alive with autumn colour. It was then that my life came rushing back to me. My eyes filled with tears and I began to sob while the dogs kept up their play with each other. All the beauty and simplicity of nature was there to enjoy. Life was bubbling up all around me and I felt ashamed of my own rejection of this incredible gift. I had started back into the light from several years in the darkness of pain.

We all have difficulties in our lives. Sometimes our problems may seem small in comparison to others but ultimately they are a large part of what defines us. Our personal story has great potential value to us if we can learn and grow from it. Sometimes it can be of value to others as well. I hope that my story can be of value to you. I am telling it to you as a way of explaining why the issue of health is so important to me. Over the past ten years I have struggled with serious injury, multiple operations, a nervous breakdown and the loss of some of those I loved most. I say this not out of any wish for sympathy or feelings of self-pity but as a framework for what I have discovered and what I hold to be of value. Compared with many I have had a very blessed life.

My greatest gift in life has been my family. I grew up in the Kinning Park district of Glasgow. My mum and dad had the challenge of raising seven children on a meagre budget. What we lacked in money was made up for in love. We lived in a two-bedroom apartment, the children all had their own beds in the bedrooms and my parents slept on a pull-down bed in the kitchen. We walked everywhere, which I'm sure served me well later in life. We never had a lunch at school. Every day we came home for a hot lunch prepared by my mum. Mum and Dad were even our main source of entertainment. Our house was filled with song, dance and games. Our small space was filled with life.

My work life started at 13 with three jobs: Sundays at the fruit and veg shop, the dairy shop after school and the hairdresser as often as she needed me. I was happy being active and making a contribution to the family. At 16 I became a secretary during the week, worked at the Citizens' Theatre in the evenings, and Saturday and Sunday back to the shop. I was a busy girl and loved it all.

My interest in health started early. Even when I was a young girl I would rather drink water than fizzy drinks, didn't eat meat, loved to exercise and eventually joined a health club when the first one opened in Glasgow. I loved to challenge my body and keep my energy up. Eventually the *Herald* newspaper hired me as a sales rep and I was flying high.

My first encounter with serious pain came on a winter night driving back from Edinburgh. A van coming in the other direction hit ice, jumped across the central reservation and slammed into me. All I remember is the flash of white lights and the searing pain as the oncoming car smashed the wing mirror through the closed window and into my head.

The car rolled over several times and the glass of the windscreen shattered and shot into my face. I was lucky to be alive, with a dislocated shoulder, black arm, 20 stitches in my head and small pieces of glass flaking off my face. It took me several months to recover. It was the first time I had experienced pain like that, but I put it aside.

During the following years I became an agent for Reebok athletic shoes. It was a perfect job for me. My passion for fitness and my love of talking to people came together. Aerobics hit big and so did athletic shoes. I was the Jane Fonda of Scotland, legwarmers, headbands and all – lord, the things we do. I got married to a lovely man and together we built an amazing business. Before I knew it, the little girl from Kinning Park was a millionaire with a home in Spain, a beautiful farm in the country, the big cars and all.

It was first class all the way. I was retired by 38 with the business sold and discovering a new love of gardening and keeping a home, doing volunteer work and leading a very active social life. Only one thing was missing: we couldn't have children. We were tested and re-tested, the doctors said there was nothing wrong, but nothing happened. I was poked and prodded and injected. Eight times I experienced IVF, but no luck.

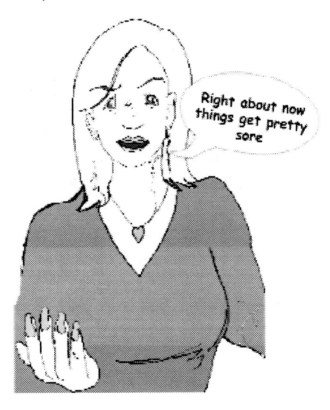

They say that life begins at 40. To me it seemed that life ended at 40. My husband gave me a beautiful gift a few days before my birthday, a frisky Irish thoroughbred horse named Cassie. He was a lovely animal, full of power, perhaps too much for me to handle. I had the cartilage removed from both of my knees because they had been torn through incorrect exercise and they were weak.

On my birthday I took Cassie for a ride. I was jumping him and my foot came out of the stirrup. He took off and I was in the air. When I hit the ground I heard a snapping sound that made me sick to my stomach. I couldn't move or breathe or speak and passed out with the shock.

Mum was at the farm and became concerned when I didn't return. She found me, called the ambulance and they took me away, strapped to a board. At the hospital it was confirmed that I had broken two vertebrae. They wanted to put me in a full body cast but I rejected it. I wanted my body to be free to heal.

When I finally stood up for the first time I felt my body was now in two pieces. The pain was horrendous, it seemed to be everywhere – my groin, my back and finally, to my surprise, my jaw. My jaw wouldn't open properly and after pouring entirely too much soup down my chin I was made a jaw brace. I couldn't eat right for years and lived on a diet of painkillers and anti-inflammatory drugs. The pain only highlighted a deeper hurt.

My life seemed hollow. It was no one's fault. It seemed that there was no colour, depth or fun any more. The sense of spirit that had nourished me as a child and teen seemed a distant dream. No matter how much I volunteered or helped others, something was missing. I was too young to be so unproductive. I had a wonderful husband, lovely friends, material wealth but I was unfulfilled. I felt riddled with guilt that I was not appreciating what I had, and prayed to God that I would find contentment. My life was coming apart, but not quite yet.

In 2001 my sister Margo was diagnosed with cancer. It was a terrible shock to everyone. We were such a close-knit family and we all hurt for her, her husband and children. As her condition continued to worsen I became aware of a catching in my breast, an aching. The family was going through so much that I didn't want to say anything and simply made an appointment to have it checked out by the same oncologist that my sister was seeing. After all the tests it was confirmed that there was an abnormality. My fear was overwhelming. I wasn't afraid of dying – I am resolved about that – it was actually the increased pain for the family that consumed me.

The day that my sister died, my marriage imploded. My friends were horrified that I was destroying what they perceived as a perfect union, and hurting a lovely man. Two days later I was in the hospital having a painful biopsy, and the removal of a piece of me. Three days after that they removed my gall bladder. They moved me into the same room my sister had been in.

Only a small group of people knew why I was in hospital. I told them it was all because of the gall bladder. I was still trying to lessen the impact of Margo's death, but the judgement of most of my friends regarding my marriage loomed largest of all. I was willing to accept the fact that I had caused pain, but it seemed that everything was disappearing into a black haze. Most of my friends rejected me, my marriage was done, my home broken and I began a slow and steady descent into the darkness.

Grieving, physical pain, rejection and self-loathing all found a ready home in me. I didn't want to live any more. The pills seemed an easy exit from a life that held no warmth or joy for me. I was found in the woods dying from an overdose, had my stomach pumped out and was sent home in limbo. It was months later when I took that walk with my dogs and some spark was reignited in me. I decided to live. It's interesting what God sends you when you make a decision. I started to study Eastern medicine and anything that was life affirming to put myself back together. Then the magnets made their arrival.

I don't believe in coincidence; right on cue, a friend introduced me to a lovely woman named Margaret Doherty who gave me a pair of magnetic insoles for my feet. When I put them in my shoes I thought my feet would catch fire. She gave me a magnetic mattress to sleep on and I woke up aching all over (this is not a usual response, by the way). I stuck with it because I knew that something important was happening, and then I noticed that my energy seemed better. Weeks later the miracle happened.

I woke in the morning and went to fix my breakfast. It was a sunny day and as I was eating my toast I realized that my jaw was pain-free. I was chewing normally and my back felt relaxed. It was stunning. It was time to rebuild my life, to pay attention and apply all that I was learning. I started walking more and exercising. I threw away the mouth brace and cleaned up my diet. The medication went in the bin and I was feeling like a new woman.

My life is so different now. I have a lovely cottage in the country; I work with people every week that I feel I can help lead a happier and healthier life. I created the Academy of Wellness to introduce health into the workplace and help empower people. Sharing this information is my passion. I know that sometimes I might be preachy, but I think it is important for us all to reclaim our health and our true potential. I have made this book simple because I like simple things. This is not a complicated issue, what I have to say either makes sense to you or it doesn't.

I know that we all want to be happy and enjoy the wonderful world we live in. When we are drowned in emotional or physical pain, we lose our compass. I have written this book to share with you what I have learned and continue to learn about the energy of life and how the mind and body are connected. As far as I can tell, life is more about learning than anything else and I continue to learn every day. I wish I had known what I know now twenty years ago. All of us have incredible gifts that we should share with each other; if I hadn't had my pain and my trials, I would just be growing my petunias.

One thing I have learned through my study and experience is this. The principles of health are not complicated. The stores are full of books that break things down scientifically and tell you details that are impressive, but the conclusions are pretty much the same. The problem is that it all gets taken apart. Health is not one thing, but everything. It has to do with everything from what we have for breakfast to how we think about life.

My guarantee to you is that if you follow the simple advice in this small book, you will improve your health. I truly believe that every day should be lived as if it were the last because it just might be; there are no guarantees. I also believe in my dream of helping and empowering people to overcome obstacles in their lives. I have taken that on as my work.

My faith is what has sustained me when all else failed. When I was in the depths of my depression, the only real thing wrong was that I lost my faith. I lost my faith in myself, in life, in God. I felt numb, a feeling of being disconnected from all whom I I knew and loved. Nature has always inspired me and even my love of that could not help me climb out of the black hole I was in until my faith was restored. I know that we can both encourage each other and bolster each other's faith or we can hold each other down. I have worked with so many wonderful people troubled by depression and poor health. It never fails to lift my spirits when I see the black cloud disappear and their eyes start to sparkle again.

There is energy, a life force that runs through us all. When we are healthy, that force bubbles up in us and connects us with each other. We have all experienced that feeling of deep connection with people we love, with nature.

That's what health is really about. Beyond the theories and the science and the surveys and studies, it all boils down to that. Health gives us the freedom to be who we really are. Life has a rhythm. There are times in our lives when we feel uplifted and times when we feel down. There comes a time when we must make a decision to make less of our life or more. My greatest joy is to experience more and my second greatest joy is to share it with you. I need to know that it works, not only for me but also for others. I live what I teach and I teach what I live. So then – that's me. Now let's open the toolbox and get to work.

CHAPTER TWO

THE WELLNESS REVOLUTION

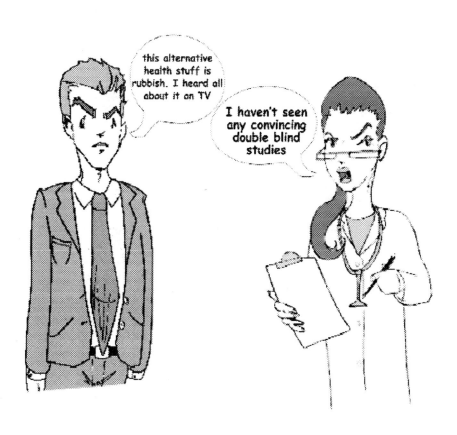

Health Service or Sickness Service

Good health has been made a mystery, and it's not. There are always things we can all do to improve our health and the only thing that holds us back are habits, the fear of change and nonsense. That is why I want to share with you my Toolbox For Healthy Living. It's simple and straightforward (like me). I know what I know because of what I've seen and experienced. We all deserve to be healthy and if we are willing to open our minds, we can achieve it.

Reclaiming our health involves creating a way of life that respects our body, mind and spirit. It is a personal journey made up of simple steps. The goal of the journey is to improve the quality of our life: to reduce stress, have more vitality and be better prepared to enjoy the world around us.

When we talk about health it invariably gets tangled up with the practice of medicine. I am not a doctor and I have no desire to be one. In fact, the whole doctor-patient thing is a big part of the problem. We talk about Health Care and Health Services, but they are never about health, they are about sickness. The money that the government spends on Health is really spent on sickness. It should be renamed the National Sickness Service.

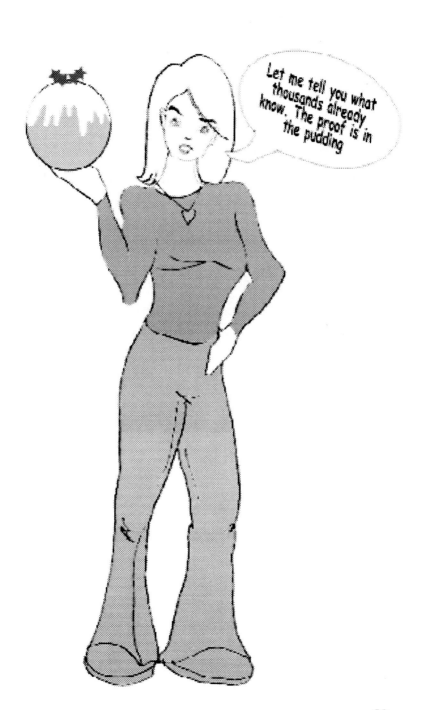

Don't get me wrong, we need a sickness service – I know from personal experience. I probably wouldn't be alive without it. Sometimes people need operations, drugs, MRIs and all of those wonderful modern techniques for dealing with serious illness or injury. We simply shouldn't confuse all of that with creating health. It's no use just muddling along till we get sick and then expecting the doctors to mend the damage. If we all wait until we get sick before we take action, we overload the doctors' surgeries, fill the hospitals, make ourselves and our families miserable and waste billions of pounds in the process. It's childish. We are all to blame. Why don't we just grow up and take care of ourselves? And we can, through one word: PREVENTION.

Here is a question for you. The bridge over a canyon collapses and cars are plunging into the abyss. There are two principle courses of action: (1) Go down into the canyon and help those who are injured; (2) Stop the traffic first, then go down and help. It is a question of priorities. Our Health Service is in the canyon doing its best, but the cars keep coming, fast and furious. Someone has to stop the traffic. The solution is not going to come from the bureaucracy – they're down in the canyon counting the cars. The solution will come from creating a critical mass of individuals, who are alert enough to look ahead, take responsibility for their health and put on the brakes. Some of those who stop will be brave enough to flag down those who are speeding by and get them to pull over too.

This health crisis exists because we are clamouring for more sickness service than can be logically provided. It came as a shock recently when it was revealed that nearly one million people fell victim to "adverse incidents" in the NHS. The same survey reported that over 2,000 deaths a year were attributed to these "adverse incidents", and that "it was widely acknowledged that there is significant under-reporting of deaths and serious incidents". An over-taxed system is a big part of the problem. It gets dangerous to be sick.

This is not only a personal issue, it is reflected in the emotional and physical effect of disease on families and society. Each year sickness costs UK employers over £11 billion. Almost 10% of the population stated that their health was "not good" in the 2001 census. One fifth are obese and one fifth report stress at work.

Look at the logic of this: heart disease and stroke are the top killers in the UK. They account for 39% of all deaths, followed by 26% for cancer and 13% for respiratory disease.

I heard on the radio the other day that by 2010 cancer will have increased by 50%. That's only four years away! The biggest health threat on the horizon is the increasing incidence of diabetes. The interesting thing is that all of these problems are largely preventable. That's right; they are diseases that we choose through the way we live.

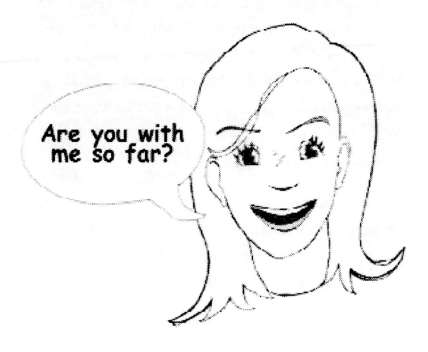

Herbs or Pills?

Let's get this out of the way and then we can get to the good stuff. There are three options to feeling better. These different approaches are: Conventional Medicine, Alternative Health Care and Wellness. The focus of conventional medicine is to treat the symptoms of illness after they have developed. The focus of the alternative medical approach is similar, with the exception that the tools used are less invasive and usually subtler.

With a Sickness Service that is overloaded, there is a tendency to use the most dramatic solutions to any problem. The closest metaphor is war: we are fighting a "war" against heart disease; the "fight" against cancer and the "battle" against diabetes. Time to haul out the big guns. Too often the first approach to any problem is the most aggressive. Any sickness becomes a case for crisis management. We contribute because taking personal action is not really an option that is presented with any encouragement.

Alternative approaches to healing include Homeopathy, Herbalism, Acupuncture, Chiropractic and a wide variety of traditional healing techniques. Lifestyle recommendations are more common with alternative health care, but that is usually not the focus of the practice. I have found many alternative approaches to be effective, including therapeutic exercise, herbal medicine, chiropractic treatment, magnetic therapy and many more. They can often stop a more serious problem from developing without more invasive treatment.

I am not a masochist, but consider this: isn't it more sensible and effective to learn something you can do for yourself, rather than run to a specialist every time there's a problem? I have learned many simple and effective things that work for me if I have a headache or stress or sore tummy. If I didn't know these things I would have to take medication that was, in reality, not needed. We get hooked into disguising symptoms and lower our sensitivity to what is really happening in our body. This is not a good thing.

Degenerative disease doesn't occur overnight. We simply have lost the ability to see what our real condition is. Our perception is clouded when it comes to seeing that we are drifting away from our potential for well being. Part of this has to do with the fact that we have split up our perception of ourselves. We don't see that our physical health, our emotions, our thoughts and our actions are all one process.

It is difficult to develop the kind of perception we need if we don't experience our life in a new way. It is really hard to describe the effect of eating sugar unless you have lived life without it for a good period of time and then had some. The same is true with water. If you drink only pure water for a month or two and then drink tap water, it tastes terrible; if you drink tap water all the time it just tastes like water.

That is one of the reasons why it is important to keep with changes in health patterns for time enough for the body to adapt. After six to eight weeks the body is getting used to a new regime; after three months you have established new habits. That is where discipline ends and being healthy is simply your way of life.

We are not educated to see that there is a whole range of symptoms that our health is declining. In fact we are taught to ignore important messages that the body sends us. We either ignore signals of physical or emotional distress, or mask the symptoms with medication. This is a dangerous system that leads us away from self-knowledge and into a "caretaker" culture. In traditional Asian medicine, everyday complaints were seen as indications of caution.

Many see tiredness as the natural state of affairs. We drink coffee or caffeinated soft drinks or take pills to perk up. Tiredness can be a symptom of many developing sicknesses from digestive complaints to problems with blood sugar. The basic symptoms occur even before you get back a troubling blood test. When a child is seen to be lethargic, everyone gets worried, but we rationalize it in an adult. If you are tired every day, unless you are working 10 hours or more, you need to take care.

The same is true with flexibility. We become inflexible when our circulation is inadequate, when our diet is toxic, when we don't get enough exercise or we have problems with our excretory system. We accept it completely.

I have had young women in their 30s tell me that they couldn't touch their toes because the were "getting old". This gets said with a combination of resignation and something approaching pride. Well, if you're getting old at 30, you better get youthening quick.

The same could be said for any number of "acceptable" problems from irritability and skin problems to headaches. The point is not that every issue can be solved at home or that individuals should be blamed for their health problems. I know all too well how a seemingly insignificant symptom can turn out to be a major problem. The idea here is to look at how we can expand our ability to care for ourselves better and how we can be more aware and responsive to our own health. We could prevent needless treatment, expense and grief. Wouldn't that be nice?

The Wellness Revolution is driven by a desire to take increased personal responsibility for health – this is the core issue. Wellness is self-generated: it is not focused on the fear of being ill but on the desire to live life to its utmost. To be happy, energetic and fit so that life can be more enjoyable and more fun. Why not?

Most of the resistance to making positive changes in our health is nothing more than habit. It is in the arena of changing personal, family and social habits that we need to focus. We really do know what needs to be done; often the controversies are merely a red herring to stop any action. Who is it that hasn't got the word that fizzy drinks are horrible for our health? Who really believes that sugar is an essential in our diet? Who doesn't know that exercise is important to health?

We could all write down at least 10 changes we could make in our life that would improve our health – we just don't do them. One of the reasons that we don't make positive changes and stick with them is that we don't see those things being done by our friends or family. We don't see information about protecting our health communicated with the same force as we see warnings about not being vaccinated. While millions of pounds are spent annually to advertise food that is a nutritional nightmare, hardly any is invested in the truly revolutionary concept of healthy living.

The sad reality is that there is almost no money spent on preventing disease or creating health, except safety programmes that tell us not to lift heavy boxes or stick our fingers in light sockets. This problem is a serious one. There is much more money spent on luring us into sickness than is spent on health.

The most money spent on advertising food is directed at children. Our children are being convinced to eat breakfast cereals that are nutritionally deficient – they would get more from eating the box! Food companies, in particular, focus advertising on the very young – they are tomorrow's consumers. We call much of the food consumed by kids "junk food" and still we buy it for them. Do we really want to feed the kids junk for dinner? The issue of taking the edge off information that could lead to better health is a priority in the food, alcohol and tobacco industries.

Disguised as independent researchers, scientists who are funded by big business regularly show up in the press to criticize responsible reports on the ill effects of products. The message is usually put out by some phoney front organization with a cute name telling us that tobacco, alcohol or some sugar-saturated product increases pleasure, reduces stress and makes our life that much better. They don't need to reveal who pays the bills. They make everyone feel better and disinclined to make any changes.

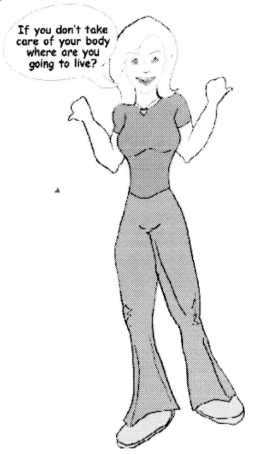

Hopefully we can move past the confusion created by Big Business, Big Pharmaceuticals and Big Medicine, and get to the truth. Creating health is not that difficult if we are willing to invest a little time and energy. Please don't wait till the last minute. It's worth the work; you might say that your life depends on it

What About Weight Loss?

Most of the interest in health over the past 15 years has been focused on weight loss. While some of this interest has been for cosmetic reasons, with everyone wanting to look like a fashion model, some has been motivated by a serious concern with health. Obesity is a very real problem, since it is a precursor of so many other serious health issues, from heart disease to diabetes.

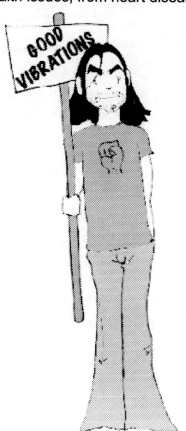

Weight loss has become a major industry with billions of pounds spent annually on products and programmes to lose weight. Here is what I have found to be true.

Most weight-loss programmes don't work in the long run because they don't emphasize being healthy.

If you are improving your health, your body will reduce (or increase) in size to its proper proportion.

Any food-based programme for weight loss without an exercise component is destined for long-term failure.

Starvation and "cleansing" or "detoxification" purges are short-term distractions unless part of a comprehensive programme.

If you follow the suggestions in this book and create a healthy lifestyle, you will find your body will seek out its natural healthy weight and stay there.

I hope that when I open the Toolbox for Well Being, you will find ideas that can help you in pursuit of a better life, regardless of your age, economic situation, education or present state of health.

There is one other difference between the Wellness Revolution and conventional health care. Much of what inspires the work done in wellness is a respect for ancient systems of understanding the body. It is interesting that centuries ago there was an understanding of how we work that can give us valuable insight into today's problems.

In India, China, Japan and other Asian countries, there was a very sophisticated appreciation of how the body worked. This system was based on recorded observations of sickness and health over centuries. What these ancients saw was that all the physical parts of the body – the bones, the organs, the tissue – comprised energy. Pretty neat. They knew what we now know – the body is a swirling sea of bioelectric energy. They called this energy by different names – Chi, Ki, Prana – but they were describing the same thing. They knew that we are part of nature and that health is achieved when that natural exchange with our environment is balanced. The study of this exchange relative to health is called Energy Medicine. When the flow of energy is blocked, we get sick. I always tell my students to keep their "valves wide open", to be open to life. They sometimes laugh but they know it's true. I used to sign off on my answering machine by saying, "Keep your valves wide open". When I started doing corporate health programmes, people said it was unprofessional. I thought it was good advice.

What About A Healthy Workplace?

Dear Marlene

I wish to convey my gratitude to you for the work you did with my staff. Your positive attitude is infectious and as such it was ideal to bring in to my legal practice. With your balanced and practical approach to nutrition and fitness you motivated my firm's staff to make changes in their lifestyle, which benefited each and every member in a different way.

Your joie de vivre is living proof that the Academy of Wellness approach works.

We all look forward to working together with you again soon.

Best Wishes,

Jeff Halliday

Senior Partner

McSherry Halliday Solicitors

In The Office – Part Two

Dear Marlene

They say laughter is the best medicine and after an afternoon with you at our offices, my team were rejuvenated.

Your down to earth approach and fun attitude certainly had an uplifting effect. I feel all of us left the room feeling more positive armed with knowledge and determined to put some of your simple tips into action, especially on how to best cope with stress. We did, and they work.

Best Wishes,

Sheila McGuigan

Human Resources Director

Martin Currie Unit Trust Ltd

Toolbox for Healthy Living

Creating a healthy life has to do with a number of factors. Each of them is important. These are the areas that have made the biggest impact on my health: **Diet, Exercise, Attitude, Relaxation and Environment**. You may think of others but these can really make the biggest immediate impact on our health. We make a mistake when we try to understand health as the result of just one thing. When anyone tells you that you can establish a healthy life by just doing one thing, run for the hills! Being healthy means we are using our full potential.

That potential will vary with each individual depending on past experiences or misfortune. There is no silver bullet, but everyone can live a life that is healthier than the one they now lead. Just a quick review of what's in the toolbox, then we can get into the practical details.

ATTITUDE

We are going to start things off with a chapter on Attitude. This is where so much of what we do begins. It may seem obvious, but if we are not clear about what we really want and why we want it, there are going to be problems. Developing a healthy attitude doesn't mean meditating for hours on the meaning of life, but it does take some reflection on our priorities and creating a plan of action that can facilitate positive change.

Many of our attitudes on health come from questionable sources with conflicting agendas. In fact, advertising is a major source of health information. This is put forward for profit not progress. We are constantly being told that particular foods are essential, based on research funded by commercial interests. Common sense is not only frowned on, it is often ridiculed, at least until it is found to be based on fact.

There are good products to buy and good things to do for healthy living, but the focus must be on making simple decisions about daily life – that's what is really important. There is no single product or action that will guarantee health, but what we do does make a difference. As far as attitude is concerned, here are some ideas I think are valuable:

Without belief in success, action is useless

Without reward, we will not act

Without a compass, we will lose our way

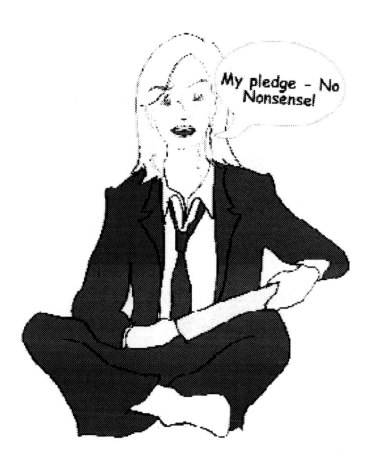

THE FOOD WE EAT

Diet is a huge issue and we are going to spend quite a bit of time on it. We are constantly being deluged with the "new best thing" in dietary advice; there is only one problem – most of what is good is not new and most of what is new is not good.

Certainly obesity is a problem, but there is more to eating well than being thin as a matchstick. Much of the information about food that we receive is based on looking only at weight. We need to change our focus and ask what kind of diet suits general health. If we have a good diet and are living a sensible life in terms of activity, we will find our weight will find its natural level. The issues of diet that are most important are:

The variety and balance of food groups

The purity of the foods we eat

Seasonal and environmental considerations

Making healthy food that tastes delicious

We are going to explore how you can get all of these factors under control so that you can have a diet that will satisfy your hunger, increase your vitality and put you in control of your weight.

EXERCISE

We all know what comes next. Get off yer butt! We have become a nation of couch potatoes. We watch over 30 hours of TV a week, but don't have the time to exercise. I'm not talking about getting your leg over your head or running three miles before breakfast. We all need to find the activity that suits our life, but we do need to find one.

It is an undeniable fact that exercise is one of the best ways to reduce stress, improve cardiovascular condition, improve diabetes, and reduce bone loss in women and the elderly. This is not theory, it's a fact. We also know that children need plenty of exercise to keep their body weight down and to improve their general health; what is our government's response? To cut down on the opportunities for kids to engage in sport!

Most people get their maximum exercise walking from their front door to the car or the bus – a distance they walk twice a day. When we are young it doesn't show up so much but as we grow older it makes a huge difference. A small amount of daily exercise can mean the difference between a healthy life and a heart attack. It's important not to wait till it's too late. We are going to talk about strengthening and stretching and give you some detailed instructions on keeping your body energized. Here are some of the items in the toolbox:

How exercise benefits the internal organs

How to increase flexibility

Exercises for work and play

Incorporating exercise into daily life

RELAXATION

Almost everyone you meet will tell you how much stress they have in their lives. Even children talk about being "stressed out". This is a fairly recent phenomenon. If this is the result of our modern way of living, then we better figure out how to get it under control or stop putting ourselves in this situation. In some people, stress is like a badge of courage. The higher the stress level we have, the more important we are. What a lot of nonsense!

We feel stressed when our body and mind feel

overloaded, overused or abused. There is nothing brave about learning to take the abuse. Stress has been associated with almost every major disease, from heart disease to cancer. When our way of life is killing us it's time to stop and think again. What's in the toolbox?

Learning to create a schedule for healthy living

Learning to calm the body and mind

Cutting down the static

Partnering for Stress-free Living

The Secret of Sleep

ENVIRONMENT

We live in two environments. One is the external environment of the natural world; the other is the enclosed environment of home, workplace or school. The external environment is our source of being. We all need to help protect it for future generations and stop its ruination. The built environment is where most of us spend our time. Whether at home or work, the air we breathe, the water we drink and the composition of these interiors affect us more than we expect.

The home and work environments are often more polluted than we think, in fact the air in many homes exceeds the levels of airborne contamination found in industrial areas. The good news is that there are things we can do to make our homes more supportive of good health. Some of them are simple common-sense actions and some are new products that can assist us in the process. In the toolbox you will find:

Making your home stress-free

Making the most of the air we breathe

What about water?

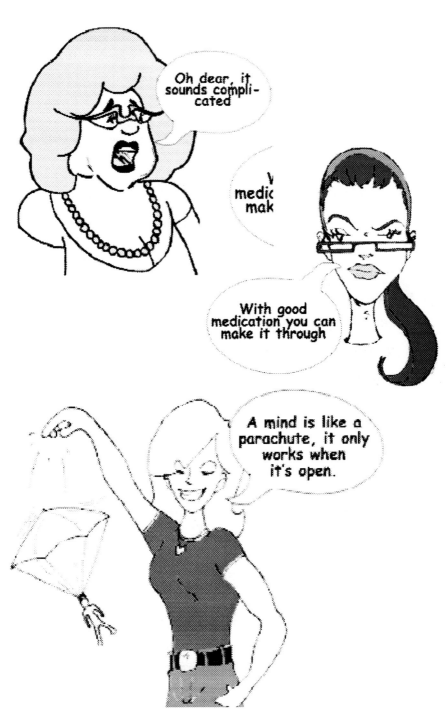

53

CHAPTER THREE

MIND OVER MATTER

Health is about freedom. Good health gives us the freedom to enjoy life more fully, to live the truth of who we really are. Much of what holds us back is nothing more than habit. We get used to the way we live our lives and so does everyone around us. When we begin to make changes, it can rock the boat, everyone gets nervous. The social pressure to be unhealthy is more overpowering than the encouragement to be healthy. This is why developing a healthy attitude is so important. Being healthy can be like swimming against the tide.

Try this. Tell your friends that you have decided to stop eating sugar or that you are going to start exercising daily, and see what happens. Make a mental note of how many people tell you that you'll never do it or that it can't make a difference. See how many of your friends are willing to share with you all the reasons they have never done it, compared with those who are supportive.

It's not that creating health is complicated – it's simple. It's just a matter of knowing what is really important to us and then making a plan to achieve it. Most of what gets in our way lies in the six inches between our ears. We are walking history books. All the information, attitudes and experiences of our life are woven into a tapestry of attitudes, habits and actions. Making changes means taking a few of those strands and giving a tug. If we don't like the pattern, we can change it.

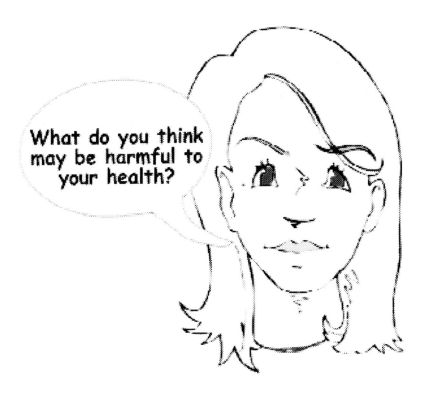

Where Do We Put Our Faith?

Don't let this put you off, but I believe in God. Not some punishing big man in the sky but more a spirit of creation and compassion. It's not important to me how others hold this thought in their minds and hearts, but it's an important part of the puzzle for me. For me, the issue of faith is fundamental to health. Not necessarily religious faith but faith in the potential we all have to improve our lot and to create happiness in our lives.

The fact that this faith has been a saving grace for me is not unique. It is well known that people of faith are able to move past the barriers of pain and despair and discover meaning in their life with greater effect. I know that when I trusted in my faith all was well, despite the pain, and when I lost my faith I began my descent into depression and suicidal limbo. I don't expect everyone or even anyone to respond in the same way, it is simply the truth of my life. I would be a liar not to say so.

When I work with clients I notice that faith in life, love of nature and appreciation of what we are given, often define personal progress in health. When our expectations are positive, our body responds to make the inner vision a reality. When the mind is plagued with negative or cynical attitudes, we are undermining our own best efforts. When started reading and studying Asian medicine, the sense of this became clearer.

One of the principles of Asian medicine is that the world is a sea of energy, call it what you will. In Chinese medicine it is called "Chi". When they talk about the body or the mind they view it all as part of one thing. Everything is constructed of the same energy that manifests itself in different forms – isn't God clever? This is not really different from what physicists say – it's all energy.

To be healthy, chi has to be balanced. We take in different forms of energy every day. We drink water, breathe air, eat food and are aware that all these different forms of energy combine within us and create our body. We take in energy from other people too. Our families, partners, workmates, all have an effect on us. Most of us can identify a person who brings us down or lifts us up simply by being in the room, and it doesn't stop there.

We take in information from newspapers, magazines, TV – all energy, all becoming part of us. Health is the act of balancing these things in terms of quality and quantity. Illness may begin in the body or the mind, in the environment or in our relationship with others. Our attitude plays a huge role in governing the effect of these influences on us.

Any disruption of the easy flow of energy within or around us can create an imbalance with wide-ranging results. The physical part of this is easy to understand. When we are in pain or when we are bodily challenged, we can easily lose our link to happiness – our attention is drawn to the hurt. When I was experiencing physical pain I was able to cope, but when so many friends turned their backs on me, the emotional hurt pushed me right over the edge. It was an extreme reaction but not unique.

Over the past fifteen years there has been increased medical research in the ways that the mind affects the body. Thoughts and feelings are all bioelectrical events. These events in the brain trigger hormone production, resulting in changes in blood chemistry and the functioning of specific organs. All of us have experienced the reality of this connection but may not have really thought about it.

This phenomenon is what makes a child get a sudden fever on the day of a big test, or a headache appears just in time to prevent attendance at a dinner with people we don't like. The symptoms are real, we are really sick, but where did it originate? In brief, people who are happy and excited about life, people who are not under stress, don't get sick as often. People who are in stable relationships and who have a spiritual outlook are healthier than those who hate their spouse or think life is just a bad joke.

If I ask people what is most important in their life, health is always in the top three. This seems logical since if we are sick all the time we don't get to enjoy anything else, not fame, family or fortune. It is interesting then that we don't seem to take our health seriously when it comes to our daily actions. This seems like a mystery but maybe it isn't.

Much of the problem has to do with misplaced faith. We may be born with a genetic tendency toward a specific disease, have a disability or suffer the effects of past illness, but we can always improve our lot. The reason we can do this is because we are miraculous in our design. No matter how you believe it happened, we are all walking miracles.

Sometimes the improvements may be small, sometimes huge, but we always have the option. Some people seem to stumble through life and live to a ripe old age without paying any attention to their health, but this is the exception and not the rule. It is important to know why we don't act on what we know. Deciding to create a healthy life is a choice we ignore at our own peril. It's quite simply a matter of where we place our faith.

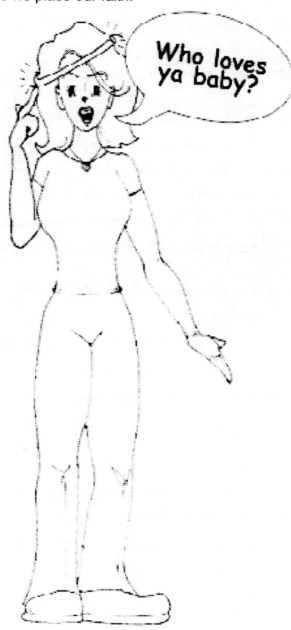

One of the reasons we don't choose wellness is that we are not fully sure that it will do any good. Our faith in our own capacity is constantly undermined. The great mass of information on health is dominated by tales of mysterious microbes, viruses and microscopic mutations to our physiology that can only be understood in a laboratory. There is next to nothing said about what we can do for ourselves. Here's one of my fantasies – the health services put out a press release that says, "You all better start taking care of yourselves or all bets are off." The reason this won't happen is we are lead to have faith in our doctors, not ourselves.

This doesn't mean that viruses or microbes don't exist. It doesn't mean that they aren't dangerous; it simply means that we need a positive attitude about our own ability to make a difference. In the past months I have heard about the possibility of Asian Bird Flu creating an epidemic. It's all over the papers and on the TV. The focus is on whether there will be a vaccine in time. I am not aware of any talk about how to create a healthier immune system, although there is plenty to say about that. There is lots of evidence that we have a greater resistance to disease with a good diet, exercise and a healthy environment. Why is this not mentioned? Much of it has to do with power.

The late Dr Robert Mendelson, the dean of medical mavericks in America, put it beautifully.

"Modern Medicine can't exist without our faith, because it is neither an art nor a science. It's a religion.

"One definition of religion identifies it as any organized effort to deal with puzzling or mysterious things we see going on in and around us. The Church of Modern Medicine deals with the most puzzling phenomena: birth, death, and all the tricks our bodies play on us and we on them. In The Golden Bough, *religion is defined as the attempt to gain the favour of powers superior to man, which is believed to direct and control the course of nature and human life.*

"If people don't spend billions of dollars on the Church of Modern Medicine in order to gain favour with the powers that direct and control human life, what do they spend it on?

"Just ask Why? enough times and sooner or later you'll reach the Chasm of Faith. Your doctor will retreat into the fact that you have no way of knowing or understanding all the wonders he has at his command. 'Just trust me'."

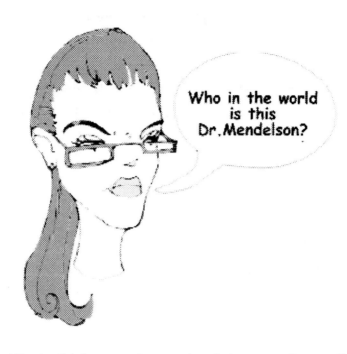

We don't take ourselves seriously because the medical system and advertising don't take us seriously. We are not empowered to make positive changes in our lives – we are disempowered. No matter how many government reports are issued, no matter how many brave souls within the ranks of the health care system speak out, the loudest message is still the same. The message is that there are things you can do to be healthy but you probably aren't strong enough or smart enough to do them. If the only faith we have is our faith in medicine, we will never take the steps needed to create our own health. The time to invest faith in medicine is when you need it, in between it is faith in ourselves and in the gifts we have been given that are essential

Our bodies are designed to be healthy. Most sickness occurs not when our bodies let us down but rather when we let down our bodies. Just think of the beauty of our immune system, our capacity to adapt to physical challenges – what a miracle. Our minds are designed to be healthy too; we just have to feed them the right food. If those around us are bound up in negativity we need ways to buffer that or remove ourselves from those influences. If our friends are not interested in making their lives full of adventure, vitality and joy – get new friends. This is all about having faith in our own intuition, having faith in our own goals and dreams and not losing our freedom.

Most people want to be "normal". We desire the cosy fabric of a close-knit social group that we belong to. The problem is – what if normal means being sick, being in debt, in a job we don't like or generally unhappy with the life we lead? This resistance to change is part of the glue that keeps us from breaking out of the pack.

Being positive is difficult when it is so fashionable to be cynical. It has almost become a way of life. Here is what my dictionary says about being a cynic:

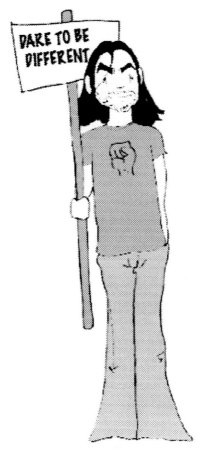

A person inclined to believe that the motives for people's actions are insincere and selfish, and who displays this belief by sneers and sarcasm.

A sneering, sarcastic person.

So then, sound like anyone you know? Some people even call themselves cynical as a label of toughness and strength. What a shame. If we live our life in that way, always suspicious of others, always determined that things would never work out, what's the point? I get this a lot in my work. When you are presenting information that challenges the status quo you do. I can tell you that pessimism is the unhealthiest of attitudes. It makes us sick and keeps us sick. There is a series of suggestions at the end of this chapter for creating a positive attitude; give them a try.

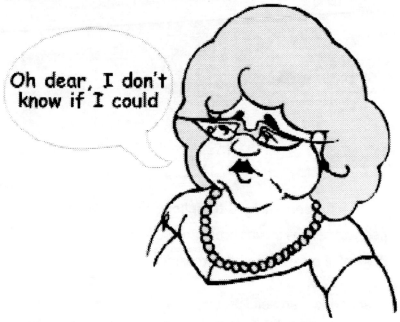

Oh dear, I don't know if I could

Creating a healthy outlook doesn't mean becoming a fanatic or increasing the stress in your life. It means that we recognize our own ability to increase control over our mind and to direct it toward our best goals. This will not stop us ever getting sick or feeling bad or being stressed out, it simply means we are using our full potential to create a vibrant life.

The term used most often to describe our discomfort with the way we live is stress. Stress is certainly a very real part of modern life. It is what happens when we are exposed to physical, emotional, spiritual or environmental challenges that we cannot cope with. Another way to say this is that stress is the result of resistance. We feel that we are supposed to be able to handle the pressures. As I said earlier, it has almost become a badge of courage.

There are countless books and seminars to instruct us on ways to run a home, be overworked and finance an increasingly expensive way of life without coming apart at the seams and running berserk through the streets. If we can do all this and not do violence to others or ourselves we are a success. We are "multi-tasking" – the mantra of the young professional. Does that make sense to you?

We are not designed to drive a car, listen to the radio, calm a child in the back seat and talk on a mobile phone at the same time. It is dangerous, the system is overloaded but we continue. We consistently override the messages sent to us by our body and mind in a manic drive to keep up with everyone else. We say that we are experiencing stress. Well of course we are. Having a healthy attitude means creating priorities that are outside this chaotic premise.

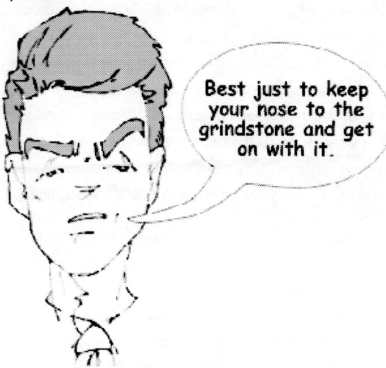

Best just to keep your nose to the grindstone and get on with it.

If someone asks us to lift their car off the ground so they can change the tyre we don't get embarrassed about not being able to do it. We don't sulk away feeling we are weak or rush out to the gym so we can build more muscle to lift it the next time. We just laugh and tell them to think again. So why do we accept increasing demands on our body and mind that distract from the real joy of life?

We all have things that absolutely must be done for our work or family but who will do them if we sacrifice our health to the god of pressure. We get used to living in a certain way and habits are formed. They are usually a way of rewarding ourselves, even if they seem strange. A person who smokes loves the way they feel when they light up, breaking the rhythm of their work and speeding up their heart rate. A person who has a glass of wine in the evening to relax may be making a wise balance; I do and I enjoy it. Someone who drinks half a bottle to wipe out the memory of the day may have a problem. We are always looking for a reward – we just want to feel good! The problem is that often our escapes make us less and less able to function in a healthy manner. Let's look in the toolbox.

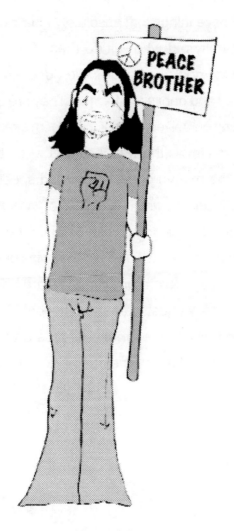

Thoughts are energy. As we grow up we start to develop ways of thinking that channel that energy in particular ways. How we channel our thoughts often has to do with how we have been educated. In fact much of our education is nothing more than getting us all to think in the same way.

This is a real problem because the world is a very complicated place with endless possibilities.

If our experiences don't conform to what we've been told are true, we filter them out. If we have only been taught to think in black and white – colour can be confusing or even threatening. Keeping our valves wide open means that we can learn to look at the world differently, see new options.

If we see the body as energy, it makes it easy to see the connection between a healthy body and a healthy mind. When we are ill the energy in the body is blocked or deficient; this deprives us of our higher faculties, the ability to think well. This was well known in Chinese and Greek medicine where various physical problems were seen as having a direct connection to our emotions.

We all know this to be true in a general sense. When you have a headache, do you relate to your friends or co-workers the same as when you are feeling well? What about if the discomfort you feel is general and chronic, could it affect your personality? When we are healthy, the energy of the mind and body flow easily and we are more adaptable, positive and clear headed. A healthy body nudges us into a positive mental outlook. That may be why people who are interested in their health are often scorned as being silly or unrealistic. Being positive is not popular.

What Frank Says

Dear Marlene

Having been diagnosed with cancer in June 2004 I felt my life had come to an end. I plummeted into the depths of despair and although the medical profession assured me that undergoing the operation to remove the tumour in my bladder had a good chance of success I was still feeling very sorry for myself. Then you enter.

You do not go in for self-pity and immediately took the situation in hand and set about organising my regime. After advising me on my nutrition and water intake you emphasised the importance of maintaining the right attitude. After listening to what you had come through I felt very humble.

It is eighteen months now since I had both my bladder and prostrate removed but thanks to you Marlene and the Doctors I am very grateful for every day I am given.

Keep up your wonderful work and go out and ignite the world with your un-stoppable enthusiasm. Your truly are contagious and I feel very blessed to have met you.

With love and gratitude

Frank Gallagher

Putting Stress By The Wayside

Dear Marlene,

Meting you not only changed my life, you transformed it. I am the MD of a busy event management company in Scotland, divorced, two children, the usual story, and therefore constantly bombarded by stress from every angle. Marlene you 'rubbed' me out and drew me back in again with amazing results. You simplified nutrition and taught me how to really look after myself. The results have been significant and my life is unrecognisable. My weight dropped dramatically even though I haven't been near a gym. Working out with you, walking, doing yoga, using my body's own weight as resistance has given me a wonderfully toned shape.

My health has improved, I feel fitter than I have ever felt. I am less stressed even though my life still involves the same stresses. When I feel I am on overload I take your advice on board and get out for a walk in the fresh air and with some deep breathing I return refreshed. I believe for the first time in my life I actually understand my body's needs.

I now sleep well and in general I am 'in control'. This is all thanks to you and the amazing work you do with Academy of Wellness. It is so simple and easy to understand and I can fit it all into my hectic lifestyle.

Thank you Marlene for teaching me about prevention.

In good health,

Sandra Light

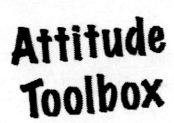

Defeating the One Million Monkeys

Imagine the mind as the sum total of all you have experienced, learned and been told. These are all influences of the past – they may or may not be true for the present or the future. If we allow old experiences to dictate our actions, we become a slave to the past. This slavery holds us back from moving into a new future.

Ask yourself how often you were told that you couldn't accomplish certain things because you were too young, too old, a woman, a man, not smart enough, not good looking etc., etc., etc. Blah Blah Blah. History is filled with men and woman who rose above difficulty to accomplish great things. These people all had one thing in common: they didn't believe the dream-stealers and the negative folks around them. They also often failed many times before success. These people are worth modelling.

If we repeat a thought enough times we start to believe it. Thoughts can become reality. If we are told something enough times we start to think it's true. If we fail at a task and are given a reasonable reason for our failure, we often embrace it. Whew! What's a poor girl to do? When we take in the myriad of excuses, rationales and unasked-for advice, we create a monkey mind.

The million monkeys are all those thoughts that confuse, conflict and contradict our intentions. Other people give us many of the monkeys. Friends, parents and spouses, everyone is happy to share their favourite mischief-maker with you. I see the monkeys in operation every day in my own life and in others. This is what happens.

When someone comes to me for personal training and health coaching, they fill out a form and we have a conversation about their health and their health goals.

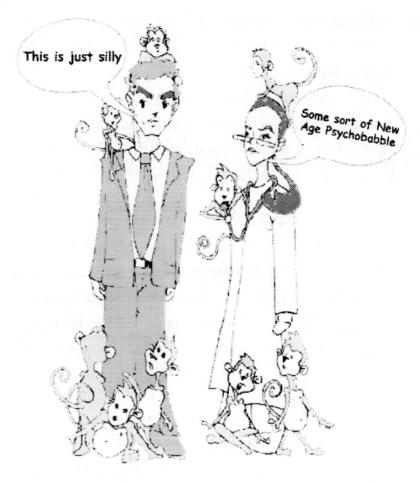

When we open the Toolbox, it is amazing how quickly the monkeys spring into action. I demonstrate a simple warm-up exercise and out pops a monkey, "Oh, I can never do that." Understand this: they have never tried to do it before and yet, "Oh, I can never do that," pops right out. They will stand and pace and grunt and groan before they even try. With time they will do it but the struggle with the monkey will make it hard for them. Some people laugh and say, "Oh boy, here goes," then they try it, they will do it quicker and it will be easier. It's all about the monkeys.

I hate to use a mechanical term for any human function but we get programmed and we all have our particular reasons why we can't do what we haven't done. I have never written a book before and I have had to deal with a lot of monkeys to get this far, both my own and other people's. I am just going to ignore them.

Over the years we come to believe these monkey thoughts are true. Guess what? If we believe them to be true, they will be. We need to recognize the monkey for what it is, and create some new programmes to run with. The bad news is that we hardly ever lose those monkeys; the good news is that they don't need to run the show. We have the ability to create new images and beliefs if we want to.

Affirmations

There are many tools to use in restructuring belief. All of them have to do with replacing old monkeys with new ones. The old beliefs were usually put in place by others or ourselves unconsciously, the new ones need to reflect conscious decisions. Some people laugh at this process as naive, some liken it to brainwashing. Why are we so afraid of our own minds? We get brainwashed every day by advertising, magazine articles and politicians. When someone else washes your brain, it often shrinks in the process. When you wash it yourself, especially on the gentle cycle, it simply becomes fresher.

One of the ways to refresh and refocus your mind is through the use of affirmations. This is a simple process of creating statements that are in alignment with our goals and repeating them to ourselves. Many years ago an American woman, Louise Hay, wrote a small book on the subject and her statement, "Every day, in every way, I'm getting better," became a buzz phrase. Some thought it was a silly thing to do in the face of serious disease. I guess they thought that, "Oh my God, I might die," or "I feel so rotten I'll probably get worse," were a better idea. You decide.

You can even read your affirmations onto a tape recorder and play them back to yourself in your car. There are some rules to doing this.

1. Make it simple.

2. Speak your affirmations with conviction.

3. Make all your statements in the present tense ("I am," not "I will").

4. Create a timeframe for your goals.

5. Have fun with this, it's not voodoo.

Here are some examples:

I only eat food that is good for my body.

Every day I learn more about my body and mind.

On or before December the 12th, 2006 I will weigh 13 stone or less.

I enjoy being healthy, having fun in my life and living my dream.

You will make up your own affirmations and change them as you go along. This need not be only something you do for physical health; it is a great way of approaching any accomplishment.

The same principles can be applied to what you see as well as what you say or hear. Write your affirmations out and keep them in your pocket or purse. When you see them or even touch them, you will be reminded of your true goals. Better still, post them where they can be seen – by your bathroom mirror or on your fridge. It's easy to forget important things in the rush of daily life; a reminder brings us back to our purpose.

On my kitchen wall I have a White Board and I write down thoughts, goals, dreams and visions. I know some people (I know who you are) think my board is total nonsense. But I have many goals there that have come true. You never see what has been erased. I know that if I don't keep my dreams alive and in my mind, I will get distracted. Here are some of the many things on it: **Lord: Give me Patience, but hurry!** (not yet affirmed); **The Academy of Wellness** (this is the name of my business – I wrote it up before it even began and it will stay there while it grows); **Marlene Macmillan's No Nonsense Guide to Healthy Living** (it might be erased by the time you read this). **We are never given a dream without also being given the power to make it come true.**

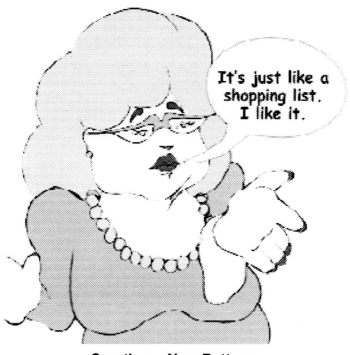

Creating a New Pattern

Our lives often become burdened with too many considerations, a jumble of needs, wants and responsibilities. If this is the case it is important to sort through them all and discover what is really most important. Excitement, exuberance, vitality and curiosity – these are the kinds of qualities we associate with health. What kinds of activities call these emotions to the fore? What is it that would make us excited to get up in the morning? What would light up our life? This is a meditation worth doing.

This doesn't mean you leave it all behind and hop on a slow boat to the South Seas. It simply means that you dream a little. You can always modify your dreams, but throwing them away or giving up on them isn't healthy. It's interesting how many people say that TV is a waste of time or that the programmes are rubbish, yet they still watch. Going on a media fast is good for the mind and soul. Simply unplug for a week or two. Try it. Use the time to read about your own body and mind or listen to music, go for a walk, meditate or just be quiet.

It is important to shake up the schedule a little to allow the mind to focus on what is missing or what needs to be cast off. Sometimes it's essential to remove ourselves from the social bustle if even for short periods of time so that we can nourish our personal needs. It's not always easy either. The demands of family, work and simply the business of life can take over. Health always involves balance.

If we are not excited about our lives we either need to change our situation or ourselves. I have seen people who have serious health problems turn their lives around with the slightest shift in behaviour. Look into your past and see if there is something that you stopped doing that used to bring you pleasure. It might be that you loved to play music, or dance or hike or paint; it could be anything that was dropped by the wayside. Rediscover your passion and it will enliven you. Health is about your whole life, how you feel, what you do, how you think.

Setting Health Targets

Start simple with the alignment of the mind and the body. Pick one or two simple health targets and stick with them. If you need to lose a lot of weight, don't shoot for ten pounds a week. Be practical, shoot for two pounds a week for five weeks and you will not only be more likely to lose the weight, but you will keep it off. Set targets that can be achieved. Once your targets are set, create your affirmations, use them and follow the guidelines to produce results. You will find many practical tools to use in the following chapters; use them. The most important part of setting health goals is the knowledge that you can meet them. The experience of success will fortify you for your next set of goals.

Allies and Saboteurs

Making changes in our way of life has its challenges and we can all use all the help we can get. Keep on the lookout for people who are also interested in creating a healthy life, and form some partnerships. Go walking together; share health goals, support each other in your adventure. We can all learn from each other and it is good to know that you are not alone in your quest for a more healthy life.

Dealing with other people's scepticism also needs to be addressed. If you are going to live a healthy life, be aware that others may not understand your actions. A good sense of humour and some humility are called for. Sharing food, drink and amusement are part of social bonding. If you start to refuse certain foods or drinks, it can be interpreted as an act of arrogance or judgement. It is your responsibility to keep it light. Being healthy doesn't mean you can't live in the real world, it also doesn't mean you run blindly with the crowd. Everyone has their own decisions to make in their own time. Having said that, there will always be the friendly saboteurs.

The friendly saboteur most commonly comes in two varieties. The first is simply concerned for your well being. When someone starts to try something new, there are questions. Is this safe; are their hidden dangers; is this some cult behaviour? The concern is genuine, there is simply an information deficit. They will be concerned that there is not enough protein in your diet, or that you might get scurvy or any number of imagined problems. They simply need information.

The second variety of saboteur is perhaps more defensive than friendly. They may feel threatened by your decisions to change routine. They are sometimes family members. They will tell you that what you are doing is nonsense, that it's dangerous, that it's anti-social. In fact, what they are doing is attempting to justify their own behaviour. After all, if what you are doing is valid, what does that say about what they do?

I have seen many men and women who were improving their health dramatically, fall by the wayside because of negative input from "friends" or a spouse. How sad.

I have had people tell me that I eat rabbit food, that my exercise regime is silly and that my affirmations are stupid. The fact that I don't need to see the doctor or that my energy levels far exceed theirs, doesn't seem to mean much; it does to me. Next year I will be fifty and I have more energy now than at forty. I must be doing something right.

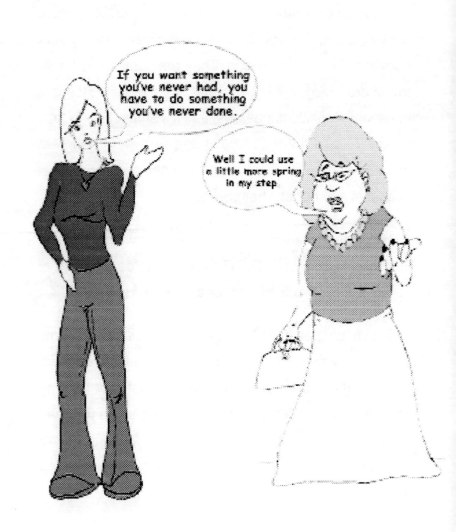

CHAPTER FOUR

WHAT WE EAT

The food we eat daily is perhaps the most important element of good health. Every chemical event in the body is dependent on your consumption of food, water and air. Food is what we are made of. Since this is true, paying attention to what we eat is essential for good health. The problem is that eating well can be a challenge in today's society.

There is a lot of concern regarding the value of different foods in a healthy diet and about the quality of the foods we eat. We are constantly being told about the newest approach to a healthy diet, so making good choices can be confusing. Every few months a new diet hits the market. We are told to avoid carbohydrates, to stay away from meat, to only eat meat, to count our calories and monitor our blood sugar – where will it end? We have tried to make life a little easier for you. One of the keys to success is to find a new attitude to food and eating that is not about dieting but about health. Enjoy your food. Nothing is more satisfying than eating tasty food that you know is doing you good. Let's take a look at some questions that are often overlooked in the great diet debate.

There are simple facts about food that shine a light on some of the problems with our modern diet. They have to do with both the types of food that humans have eaten over the centuries and the quality of the foods we eat today. Our capacity to digest and process foods is a reflection of our past eating habits. This is true of all creatures. Much of the character of any animal is dictated by its eating habits.

Our digestive system is designed to be more efficient with some foods than with others. Our particular nutritional needs are dictated not only by our human history but also by the environment we live in, the activities we pursue and our culture. If we look at human society over the centuries we see that there are many clues to what a healthy diet might look like.

The highest concentration of human life has always been in those areas with a moderate climate. It is in these areas that farming developed. With the exception of environments with poor soil, these people ate a diet that was startlingly similar. Cereal grains and beans, foods that could be stored year round, became the principle food. Seasonal vegetables and fruits were used as the secondary foods, usually in the season of growth or dried for later use. The use of milk, cheese and other dairy foods were used mostly to supplement the diet along with fish, fowl or wild game, depending on the region.

What is interesting here is that this kind of diet, with the emphasis on complex carbohydrates, vegetable protein and fresh vegetables, is the one that seems best suited for human health. The people who argue with that are generally trying to sell you a new dietary product or stop you from buying prepared foods. We are omnivores, we can utilize a wide variety of foods, if needed, but the term "needed" is important here. There have been many studies of large populations (the only ones that count in nutrition) which have shown that this type of diet is best for the reduction of heart disease, cancer and many of the diseases that plague modern society.

We associate wholegrain diets with countries in Asia and Africa, but as recently as the early 1800s most people in Western countries ate a diet that was not that different. Porridge, wholemeal breads, peas and other beans were food for the common people. Meat, fish and fowl were used sparingly. Most cattle were used for dairy products. The diseases that were most responsible for death were caused by poor hygiene, not diet. In today's society, diet is implicated in the high incidence of heart disease, most cancers, diabetes and a wide range of health problems in adults and children.

Human beings can eat a very diverse diet, but there are clues in our physiology that give us some indications what this really means. The mouth is the first place to look. Every creature on the planet has a mouth that is suited to the foods that have been eaten as it developed.

We have a small mouth (well, some people do) that is blessed with cheeks. Cheeks usually indicate that whatever we ate in our evolution is held in the mouth when we eat and not swallowed immediately. Dogs, lions and wolves have no cheeks – it's tear and swallow. You don't need cheeks for meat.

We also have a huge preponderance of molars and premolars. These teeth are for grinding. When you look into the mouth of a cow, you will see lots of grinding teeth (not that you would want to look into a cow's mouth). We have four canine teeth, for tearing, and in front, ten incisors for cutting. What do you think? Is this a coincidence or does it tell us something? It would appear that in the past we ate a diet that was heavy on foods that had to be ground, quite a few foods that had to be cut and some foods that needed to be torn. We grind grain, beans, nuts and seeds. We cut vegetables and we tear meat.

There are also certain foods that are more easily digested than others. Some foods we eat actually start digestion in the mouth so that they can be utilized completely. These foods need to be chewed well and as we chew (if we chew) they begin to break down. These foods are the more complex forms of carbohydrates, specifically whole grains. The sugars in complex carbohydrates begin to be released when we chew, making them sweet to the taste. They are also stored more efficiently in the body so that they can be used when we need them. We will talk about these foods later but it should be noted that rice, barley, oats, millet, wheat and maize were the principle foods in most regions of the world where agriculture existed.

Where the climate or the environment dictated, we adapted to a different way of eating. Northern hunters or people who lived in areas not suited to agriculture, adopted diets that were appropriate. An Eskimo needs a high-fat diet; he lives in an environment that demands it. The cold winter demands the insulation that the fat provides. We have to use our common sense. Ask what the result would be if a person working in a heated office ate the same amount of fat without the extreme physical challenges? The answer is Heart Attack.

We have also introduced new chemical compounds into our diets in the form of food additives. In the years since World War Two, there have been thousands of new additives approved for use. Some of these are for preservation, but the main reason is to make food taste, feel, smell and look better than it really is. This chemical feast is made up of substances previously unknown in the human diet. Some of these chemicals are known to cause cancer in higher doses. They have no nutritional value and they are toxic, the body doesn't know what to do with them. They can be stored in fatty tissue and build up there. Who says this is OK? - The food industry.

Pre-prepared foods are designed to make you like them. This is done by chemically manipulating the smells and tastes of the products. You would not eat them otherwise. Chemical aromas, which are devised to be released as gas when you eat them, generate much of the flavour, particularly in fast foods. It is the smell that really gets us going. The strawberry flavour used in some products is manufactured containing: amyl valerate, anethol, anisyl formate, benzyl acetate, benzyl isobutyrate, butyric acid, cinnamyl isobutyrate, cinnamyl valerate, chgnac essential oil, diacetyl, dipropyl ketone and almost thirty other ingredients.[i] What does that have to do with strawberries? Would you eat it if all the ingredients were listed separately?

These are the kinds of chemical cocktails that fall under the heading "flavouring agents". You don't need to be given all this information on food packages because it wouldn't fit! Anyway you don't need to worry, you don't need to ask questions, all you need to do is keep on buying it.

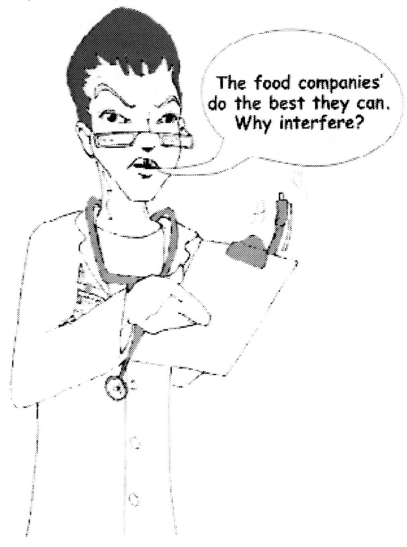

The truth is that over time our bodies have become most effective at processing certain nutrients. That is not difficult to understand, this is the same with all animals. When we change the kinds of foods we eat dramatically, the body gets confused. The most dramatic changes in our food have happened very recently, much of it immediately after World War Two. As we have changed the quality of our foods, we have seen a rapid rise in degenerative disease. This rise is directly associated with the foods we eat.

Every major scientific study, every major association concerned with the prevention of disease (including obesity) agrees on several dietary facts.

A low-fibre diet contributes to heart disease and many cancers.

A diet high in fat and cholesterol (found in fatty meats and dairy foods) contributes to heart disease.

High sugar consumption contributes to obesity and diabetes.

Nitrates (found in processed meats and fish) contribute to cancer.

High sodium contributes to hypertension.

Let's add in some additional information that is gaining credibility every year.

Contamination of the food supply with chemicals used in growing foods is harmful to general health and may contribute to a variety of health problems, particularly in children.

Increased consumption of caffeine contributes to problems with the stomach, adrenals and nervous system.

Increased sugar consumption contributes to behavioural problems in children as well as adults.

Excessive use of alcohol causes problems with the liver, kidneys and nervous system.

What does this look like to you? From my point of view this looks like the diet that most people in the UK and America consume. The diet that makes us sick is the one we eat. It is a diet based around meat, a few potatoes, very few vegetables or fruit, lots of sugar desserts and loads of fat. This especially looks like a fast-food diet. These facts are no secret, you probably already knew them.

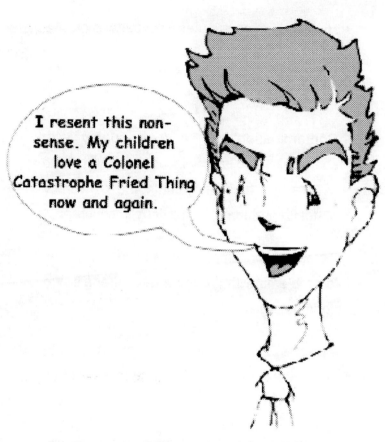

I resent this nonsense. My children love a Colonel Catastrophe Fried Thing now and again.

If you want to get the full impact of this diet you need look no further than my native Scotland. Out of the twenty-five least healthy neighbourhoods in the UK, twenty-two are in Scotland. An American firm, Caci, developed the system used to measure this. They take into account tobacco use, alcohol consumption, weight and exercise. Many will point to these locations and say it has to do with poverty, but this is not the only factor.

Even among the most affluent Scottish males, the expectancy for a healthy life is only 62. Oh, we will point to the life expectancy of 16 years beyond this but that means 16 years of sickness and medical care before they die. This makes me sad. All of Scotland lags behind national averages in well being. We all know that smoking and excessive alcohol use lower life expectancy, but the diet piece is often left out of the equation. What do we expect when we look at the food we eat? Importantly, what do we say to the next generation who have to pay for a generation of seriously ill adults while their own health deteriorates?

The good news is that we do know what a good diet looks like. Again, most authorities who base their opinions on real research rather than trying to pander to popular taste or commercial interests agree. Isn't that nice?

A diet high in soluble fibre is good for the digestive system and helps prevent heart disease and some cancers.

A diet rich in antioxidants (found in fruits, vegetables and green tea) helps promote internal repair and protect the body from cancer and other serious disease.

A diet with moderate to low consumption of

salt and nitrites helps to prevent heart disease.

Restricting fatty meat and dairy food helps reduce heart disease and some cancers.

A Macrobiotic Option

The macrobiotic diet, originally promoted by the Japanese philosopher George Oshawa and popularized in the West by Michio Kushi, comes closest to defining how to eat a balanced diet that reflects the above statements. The term "macrobiotic" means "large life" or living to our full potential.

I have found this approach to eating very helpful, even though I don't follow it rigidly on a daily basis. The Standard Macrobiotic Diet uses a simple approach of looking at daily food consumption in terms of percentages eaten in food groups during the course of a day. The percentages are an estimate and are given as a guideline. Even though there are specific guidelines for different health problems in many macrobiotic books, it is the Standard Diet that is of most interest. It is amazing how much it conforms to what is known about a healthy diet.

Oshawa was an early proponent of the importance of maintaining the acid-alkaline balance in the body. Since then many have focused on this issue as one of the primary considerations in creating a healthy diet. This is logical since one of the most important functions of the organs is to maintain a very narrow range of Ph. This is the relationship between alkaline and acidity in the body. If the balance gets off even a little bit we begin to become sick. An acid condition is essential for most disease processes, including cancer.

If our diet is filled with foods that produce an acidic condition we are constantly working to redress this imbalance. Oshawa recommended that the best foods to eat for most people were ones that gave the body the least work to do in creating the proper balance. The diet was based on grains, vegetables and beans. He noticed that some of the tropical foods that were becoming more popular in the West (citrus fruits, sugar, coffee, bananas, tomato and nightshade vegetables), coupled with heavy consumption of meat, had a tendency to tip the scales toward acidic conditions. He saw this way of eating as stretching the body's ability to make balance to the breaking point. His prediction that these foods would cause an epidemic of cancer in the West was sadly accurate.

Macrobiotics is not a diet but an approach to choosing food. It is recommended that individuals take into account their environment, activity levels, general health to make choices that fit their health goals. It is also important to eat within the seasonal cycles. Much of this is based on traditional Asian concepts of balance. I'm going to share with you what I know about this way of eating in the next chapter.

Alison's Big Day

Dear Marlene

Having suffered for years battling with my weight, numerous visits to GP's, specialists, dieticians, hypnotists and sporadic exercise routines, all of which had little or no effect I was at the point of sheer desperation and thoughts of extreme surgery.

For years I have attended Doctors, eventually diagnosed as having an under active thyroid but still finding it impossible to shift the weight after being given medication. Having been made to feel as though I was a secret biscuit eater by several medical personnel as they asked me what I ate during the day, and even asked by some if I perhaps was sleep walking and possibly eating while roaming the house.!!

All that changed when I decided to enlist the help of you Marlene. Working on a one to one basis to finally take hold of my life and see an end to the excess weight I carried and the unhappiness that went with being over weight. I thought instead of trying to battle to lose the bulge with endless diet clubs, who can't offer any alternative advice if things are not working – which they often didn't for me, I would work with you to understand just how my body was working or not as the case may be.

My first call to you put me totally at ease with your cheerful pleasant voice. Your friendly and positive attitude kept me lifted until my appointment. On that first day instead of feeling like a fat blob with no hope I was greeted like an old friend. I felt totally inspired and knew instantly we would get on. I knew that failure was not going to be an option.

I'll never forget the first time you took me on a walk in the weighted trainers to assess my fitness levels. Off we went at a fair rate and within a few minutes I thought the nightmare would never end. Your words of encouragement and chatter on the route back took me past the shaking legs and lungs that were fit to burst.

After years of thinking I was fairly fit, I found out that I was certainly not. We returned to your studio to do some yoga! With my aching body but raised spirits I left the studio on a complete high.

It only took a couple of weeks to realise just how much my fitness levels had increased and I was not dreading the walk or the yoga. I have only been working with you for a few months but feel huge benefits in many ways. I now understand foods and how they work in my body, which has encouraged me to stick to my diet. I feel that I am far more sensitive to certain food groups and feel much better about them being eliminated from my diet.

This along with the regular exercise has helped me build up my self-esteem so I feel much healthier, look leaner and have an overall better opinion of myself. I am delighted with my continued weight loss every week and as my confidence grows and my goals get closer I will still continue to work with you. Your attitude is infectious with constant words of encouragement and inspiration. I have discovered muscles that I never knew I had and perform Yoga Asanas that would have taken me years to perfect. Marlene you are an amazing woman. Thank you.

Alison Durie

Food Craving Toolbox

The single thing that limits our ability to make changes in our diet is HABIT. When we attempt to make changes, our habits come to the fore. It is important to be able to recognize what kind of habit is creating the resistance so that we can be successful in our quest for better health. Remember those monkeys from a few chapters ago? Under the heading of food cravings live many, many monkeys. The urges we have for particular foods all have their purpose. Our cravings are real. If we try to rely on discipline or willpower to succeed, we are setting ourselves up for failure. Remember, monkeys are most strong when we don't know that they are there. Here are some of the more common sources for food cravings and some ideas for dealing with them.

Biological Cravings. This may seem obvious but many who try and fail to change their diet aren't respecting their body's cry for nourishment. Biological cravings are real events; the body needs a nutrient and communicates it through a craving. There is only one problem. We are the ones who have given our body the vocabulary for communication. The body really requires a double cheeseburger. You may want one but the body doesn't. What the body may need is more protein, more heat. If the way the body has got used to getting a particular nutrient in a particular way, that's what you will crave. You can change this by re-educating your body to recognize new foods, new sources of energy and nourishment.

Be ready for a revolution. Biological cravings bring out the child in us all. When we want our Kit Kat bar, we want it now. It will take a while before you can override the Kit Kat Craving with a piece of fruit and not deal with a very childish monkey. Trust me, it will happen.

The trick is to use the substitutions in the next chapter and simply keep reminding yourself of your health goals.

Sensorial Cravings Sometimes people talk about a particular food and you wonder if you should leave the room. It's so private; it's so passionate, almost sexy. Sensorial pleasures can be very important, particularly

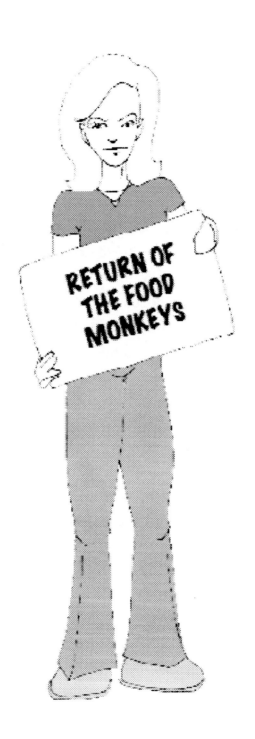

food pleasures; after all, the food gives pleasure and doesn't talk back (most of the time, anyway). There is no reason that healthy food needs to be bland and boring. The sensory connection to foods normally has to do with smell, texture or taste. They are sometimes linked with emotional cravings but not always.

The key to changing sensorial cravings is usually found in the kitchen. It is important to find foods that have textures, tastes and smells that are pleasing. It is also important that you introduce new foods so that you can expand the palette of your tastes. You may remember foods that you couldn't eat as a child but that you learned to love as an adult – same thing. Be sure to be aware of the monkeys that surround this issue – monkeys don't like to change.

Emotional Cravings. We all know the scene where the singleton curls up on the couch with a pint of ice cream. Food is often a replacement for anything missing in our lives. It can be relaxation, stimulation, anxiety, boredom or sex but when emptiness shows up we often try and fill it with food. I have yet to hear someone say, "I was so bored I ate some grapes." No, emotional eating demands some drama, it demands sensory overload, it demands chocolate!

Emotional eating is one reason why so many people

have trouble with their weight. How many times have you been bored and looked in the refrigerator for some stimulation? The interesting thing is that if there's nothing there you might check back again later and see if something interesting has magically materialized while you were gone. This pattern is most common with late-night eaters.

This kind of pattern can be developed when we are young and given food as a reward or distraction. Isn't it interesting how often we see parents give a child snack food just to shut them up? Little Bobby or Betty throws a tantrum and a sweetie gets shoved in their mouth. What's the real lesson here? The solution is to develop another strategy, fill the emotional need with something new, particularly something that requires physical activity or occupies our attention or creativity.

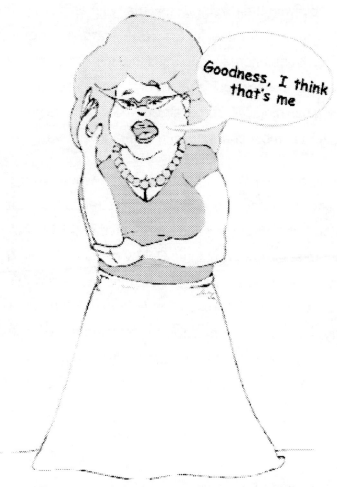

When the craving monkey leads us to the fridge, why not take it out for a walk instead. Turn off the TV and do some stretching exercises, some yoga or read a book. I have noticed that some of my clients break the snack habit when they take up a new hobby. Idle hands are the food monkeys' playground.

Cultural Cravings. All of us grow up in family and cultural environments. Food is an important part of these settings whether we know it or not. Some people completely reject the foods of their youth and become more worldly in their tastes as an act of rebellion or rejection of their culture or family. Some people get completely locked into early eating patterns. Some kind of a balance is usually called for. The process of freeing ourselves from a restrictive or counterproductive diet is not a wholesale rejection of place or family.

It may be that by changing ingredients and cooking styles, dishes that are culturally familiar can be made healthy. No reason why substitution can't work well. We will explore some recipe ideas later in the book.

When we look closely we can see that there was often a reason why certain foods were eaten and the original need has disappeared. Here in Scotland, the weather is wet and cold for much of the year. If we go back one hundred years, we see that most people had little money and that houses were often cold. The diet started to feature increased consumption of fat in any form. Fatty foods became the norm, just to keep warm. Well, the heat is on now, the toilets are inside and so are we, but the fat marches on. Time to re-evaluate. Time to eat a really modern diet, one not dictated by food producers but by common sense.

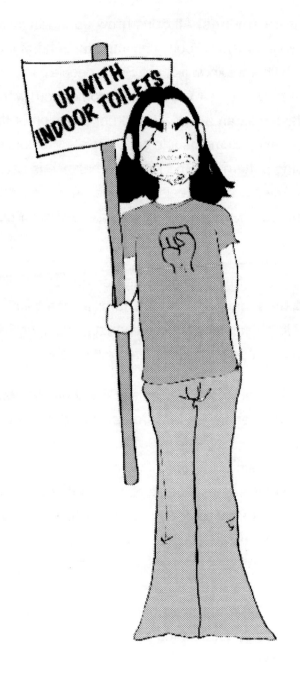

CHAPTER FIVE

CREATING A BALANCED DIET

I want to simplify the diet issue for you. You don't have to be a nutritionist to understand nutrition. The world of biochemistry is fascinating but not a pressing issue when you want to decide what's for dinner. If we look to the traditional Asian approach to food science we see that thousands of years ago, men and women had worked out the principles of healthy eating. What is really interesting is that their conclusions are a mirror image of those reached by modern researchers. Some of you might be disappointed that it's so simple. The main topics I want to share with you in this chapter are the importance of the different food groups and how they work together.

Cereal Grains – The Foundation

One idea that helps create a healthy diet is the choice of a principle food. This is a food that your whole diet is built around. The cereal grains perfectly fit this role. Their ability to complement other foods is well known. They combine nutritionally with a wide variety of healthy foods to deliver the maximum nutritional impact. Did you ever wonder why the phrase for sitting down to eat is, "having a meal"? Why is it that "Give us this day our daily bread" is not, "Give us this day our slab of meat"? Grain is a special food in human history.

The controversy over carbohydrates generally overlooks an important fact: there are refined and unrefined varieties. Refined carbohydrates are whole cereal grains that have been milled, with most of the essential nutrients removed along with the valuable fibre. These foods include white bread, cookies and other white flour products as well as refined sugars. For many people, refined carbohydrates are a major food group. While these foods may be valuable as comfort foods or for occasional use, they are not foods that make a valuable contribution to good health.

One of the most popular dietary fads of recent times has included the elimination of carbohydrates. Since most people only eat refined carbohydrates, taking these foods out of their diets will produce weight loss. They could have lost the same weight, and had more long-term success, by simply using whole grains in place of the cookies, white rice, bread and other refined products. Store shelves are now filled with "low carb" foods – great for marketing, bad for health.

Refined carbohydrates, such as sugar, give a sudden rush of energy whether we need it or not. These energy rushes from the sugar in fizzy drinks, sweets and similar junk food products are not only short-lived, we feel we need more after the rush is over. We become enslaved to extreme highs followed by a slump of energy. If you don't think sugar is addictive, wait till you eliminate it and see what happens. Did you ever notice that children with a sweet tooth only act up when they want sweeties? We see baby sugar addicts going through withdrawal in supermarkets all over the world in front of the sweet counter. Do they ever throw a fit in the vegetable section?

The value of complex carbohydrates in the human diet is that they provide a steady supply of energy that is released according to the body's needs. Complex carbohydrates can achieve this simply because they have the range of nutrients necessary to accompany the use of the sugars. To metabolize simple sugars the body has to raid its stores of minerals and vitamins. It is not unfair to say that refined sugar has a negative nutritional value; it takes away more than it contributes.

Grains are the staff of life. They have been used for centuries by people from Asia to Africa, Europe to the Americas, as the basis of a healthy diet. Brown rice and other wholegrains such as **oats, millet, buckwheat, quinoa and barley** are nutritionally better than white rice because they retain fibre and a range of B vitamins and minerals. Choose plenty of wholegrain foods and few made with white flour. **Wholemeal and wholegrain bread and pasta** contain **wholegrains** that are rich in fibre, vitamins, minerals and antioxidants.

Partially refined products such as **bulgur and couscous,** can be used as ingredients for salads, casseroles, soups and vegetarian recipes.

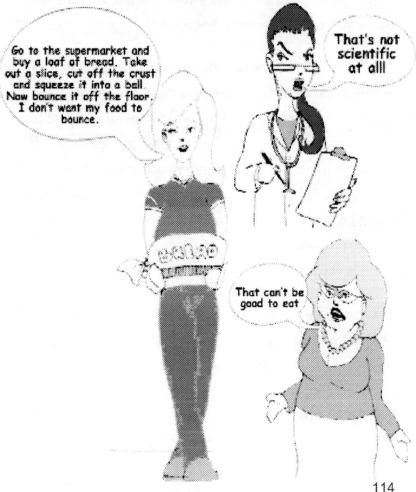

Vegetables – The Perfect Complement

Next to whole grains, fresh vegetables are the single food group that is most underused in the modern diet. They are storehouses of nutrients and micronutrients. It is important that we eat a wide range of vegetables with our meals to get the maximum benefits. They have been shown to reduce the incidence of many illnesses and have a pronounced influence in general health improvement.

Vegetables are our most important source of vitamins, those essential biochemicals for healthy functioning. Every year scientists uncover more evidence that people who eat more vegetables have a higher resistance to disease. Recent studies at Georgetown University in America indicate that natural micronutrients in some vegetables, such as broccoli and cabbage, seem to repair damaged DNA. This fits right in with what has been discovered concerning antioxidants. No mystery here. When the use of whole grains and vegetables decline, cancer rates increase.

Vegetables and fruits are the best source of antioxidants, the nutrients most associated with cell protection. Vitamins A, C and E are among the antioxidants. Listen to what Dr Richard Cutler, Director of Anti-Aging Research at the National Institute of Health in America has to say about them. "The level of antioxidants in the body is a good measure of health directly and is proportional to our vitality, resistance to disease and longevity." Wow. Did you hear that? Vitality, longevity – sign me up!

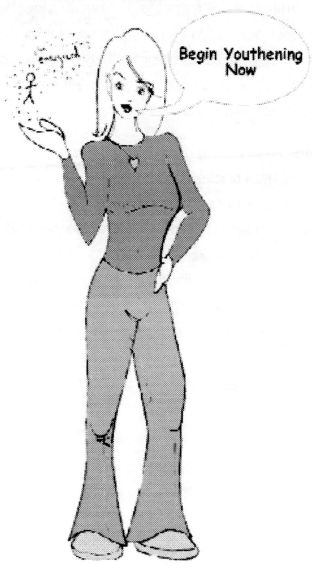

The reason we need antioxidants is because they help repair the damage done by free radicals. Sounds like a science-fiction movie: the Antioxidants putting up the good fight against the ravages of the dreaded Free Radicals. Well, it's true. Free radicals are toxic substances that occur in the body when it is under stress, or exposed to smoke, air pollution, bad diet, food additives and poor hydration. There is a constant struggle in the body to repair the damage done by free radicals and to protect the cell from damage. The damage from free radicals is reflected in premature ageing, low immune response and many chronic diseases. Free radicals can lead to cell death. Just like rust on a car, oxidation is rust in our bodies.

The cells of the body are made up of molecules and inside the molecules are electrons. Free radicals are created when molecules become unstable through the loss of an electron. In this condition they try to attack the molecules in other cells and steal an extra electron. If the little devils get out of hand, you start to lose vitality, have diminished immune function and begin ageing. This is why we are always urged to have up to five helpings of vegetables or fruit a day. Antioxidants are also found in seeds, legumes, nuts, grains, soy products and green tea.

Foods that are highly coloured are rich in antioxidants. Red, yellow, orange and green foods are readily found among the vegetables and fruits in our local shops. We should have richly coloured foods in our shopping basket when we pay and not just brightly coloured wrappers.

Vegetables are also our primary source of Enzymes. Enzymes are the foundation of energy and the life force in all living things. They are the biological keys that unlock the potential of chemical activity in the body. Without enzymes, seeds would not sprout, fruit would not ripen, leaves would not change colour and you would not exist. Enzymes are responsible for building, detoxifying and healing your body. They are the force that allows your body to digest and absorb food. Enzymes also regulate tens of thousands of other biochemical functions that take place every day in your body. These functions include breathing, growing, smelling, tasting, stimulating nerves, defending your body against disease, regulating hormones and building organs, glands and tissues. Even your thinking involves enzymes.

We manufacture enzymes in the body but they are also found in raw foods and in the sprouts of seeds and grains. The greater the challenge on the digestive system the more enzymes we need. With the increased challenge to our system through stress and exposure to environmental toxins, there is a good case to be made for increased consumption of some raw food in the diet as well as possible supplementation.

If we want to make sure that we are getting adequate nutritional support we should be having at least three to four kinds of vegetables a day. Both lunch and dinner should have healthy portions of vegetables as well as a wholegrain product. Salads and raw vegetables are perfect foods to use for snacks and as a source for some of the nutrients that are destroyed by cooking. But don't have all your vegetables raw. Depending on the time of year and your climate, cooking is important as an aide to digestion and for bringing out the flavour if done correctly. One of the reasons that many people don't eat vegetables is that the taste has been cooked out of them. We have included some cooking hints in the next chapter.

THE PROTEIN PARADOX

There is no question that the most emotionally charged issue in diet is what to do about meat. The subject is complicated because there is a moral matter involved as well as a nutritional one. As a child I never really liked red meat, but ate it. As an adult I have found huge resistance from others as I made the decision to stop eating red meat and then fowl as well. I felt like an alcoholic in a roomful of boozers. If I went out to dinner and people had cooked a roast or a chicken and I just ate the vegetables, it was construed as an insult or a betrayal of some social convention.

The whole "to meat or not to meat" question really brings out the food monkeys in many people. Men in particular seem to have this idea that if they don't eat meat they will lose their masculinity. Here's a little newsflash – if men ate a more heart-healthy diet, there would be a big dip in Viagra sales; remember, it's all about circulation. Have no fear of Tofu men – tofu is your friend.

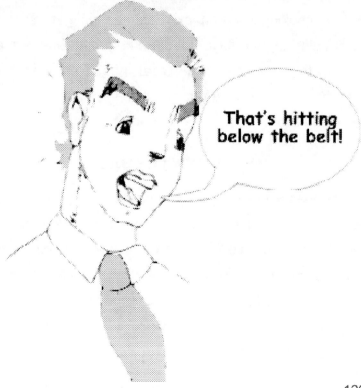

Right now I eat fish very rarely and could easily see myself becoming a vegetarian one-day. The ethical issue is definitely there for me. Sheep and cows roam the fields all around me. I watch them through the year and love to see the young ones in the spring. I know that I'll probably get a letter or two from people who see the hypocrisy of my fish eating; I'll work it out.

We need protein in our diet, it provides the basic building blocks for soft tissue in the body. We are made of water and protein. Protein comes ready-made or in a handy Do-It-Yourself kit. Ready-made is meat, the animal has done all the work and made the protein. This ready-made protein has a number of setbacks. Firstly, we have to break down the animal protein to use it, and second, it usually comes along with a fair amount of fat.

Meat is not all that easy to digest. It has to stay in the gut for a long time and decomposes leaving quite a bit of toxic material in its wake. Ever notice that carnivores usually gorge themselves and then go to sleep? It takes a good while for the energy of the meat to be released and used. Watch what happens next holiday when the meat-eaters unloosen their belts.

Using dairy foods and eggs as a primary source of protein creates many of the same problems. It is best to limit these foods to occasional use. One of the things I have noticed with many of my clients is that if they cut the dairy food out of their diets they notice nothing but positive results. The most common thing they notice is that any problems with mucus or sinus conditions improve. This is especially true with children. I have talked with many parents who noticed that inner-ear problems with their children were connected to dairy consumption. There are many good sources of calcium, including seeds, nuts and some dark green vegetables.

The types of fats in meat are generally unhealthy if eaten in excess. They are saturated fats that increase the possibility of heart disease at the very least. Some studies implicate the high meat, high fat diet with a variety of degenerative diseases. If we are concerned with where we get our protein, then DIY is the way to go.

Do-it-yourself protein is made from a combination of grains, beans, vegetables and seeds. The benefits of DIY protein are that it is easier to break down and absorb as well as the fact that it produces more elastic muscle tissue. All the amino acids we need to make healthy tissue are found in vegetable sources if we combine them well. The good news is that you don't need a chemist in the kitchen to do it. Just use vegetables in combination with grains and beans, use some seeds as a garnish and you're in business.

If you are going to use animal protein or are going to move toward a vegetarian diet, using the easiest to digest is best. Fish is preferable, fowl comes next and mammal meat is the last choice. Beans and pulses, including lentils, chickpeas and soy, are a virtually fat-free source of protein, rich in soluble fibre that helps to lower cholesterol.

Asian protein foods, such as Miso, Tofu and Tempeh are probably new to you but are good to experiment with. These foods come from the vegetarian cultures of the Far East and are all fermented forms of the soybean. Take a look at the recipes in the next chapter.

FATS AND OILS

Fats are essential for the proper maintenance of the body, including the brain. The problem is that we get too much of the wrong kind of fats. Fats comprise saturated, monosaturated and polyunsaturated fats. The Western diet mostly comprises the first two, saturated and monosaturated; these are the ones that can kill you. Wouldn't you know it?

People in Britain and America eat more than twice as much fat as the body requires. We have limited our intake of fats to meat, cheese, milk, butter and the artery-clogging stuff they put in snack foods. We have been ignoring that all the essential nutrients that we need are available in much better forms in natural vegetable, seed and nut oils.

The best way to get the balance of oil-based nutrients we need is by using cold-pressed vegetable oils, such as olive oil, sesame oil and flax seed oil. These oils can be used in cooking or as a dressing for salads. We can also use seeds. Pumpkin seeds, sesame seeds and sunflower seeds are a healthy source of oils and can be used as a snack, or a garnish. Avocados contain healthier monounsaturated oil, as well as antioxidant-boosting vitamin E.

Nuts such as almonds, Brazil nuts and walnuts contain both unsaturated omega-3 oils and monounsaturated fatty acids. Mixing seeds and nuts as a snack is also a good way of getting what you need.

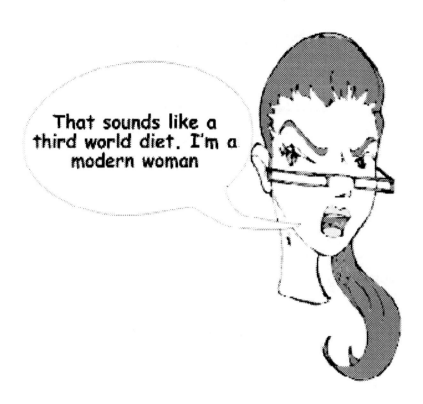

That sounds like a
third world diet. I'm a
modern woman

Just a word here about an issue that often gets passed over. Animals today are exposed to a wide range of toxic substances that are used in modern agriculture and farming. Herbicides, pesticides, fertilizers and other chemicals abound on the modern farm. It has also become normal to use hormones in the raising of animals to increase growth. Guess which part of the animal these substances stick to with ease? You got it: fat tissue.

FRUIT – HOW SWEET IT IS

Most of what has been said about fresh vegetables can be repeated for fruit with one exception – fruit is sweet. The fresh taste and sweetness of fruit are a real bonus to these important foods. Fruits can be seen as the gift to the sweet tooth and as a relaxing influence in the diet.

The sweet taste is an important one; it gives us a great deal of pleasure. When we eat a diet that is filled with simple sugars, we often lose the ability to appreciate the sweetness in natural foods. Fruits are usually eaten raw and so the antioxidants and enzymes they contain reach us in an undiluted form. They are rich in vitamins that help us build a strong immune system and ward off disease if they are used in moderation.

I am going to talk about eating with the seasons, but it is important to note that fruit is best eaten in or near its season of growth. Use this guideline if it is a food that spoils quickly; try and eat it as fresh as possible. Modern transportation has given us the ability to import fruits and vegetables from great distances. This seldom makes sense from an economic or health viewpoint. When we are eating foods that are regionally raised, we are supporting local producers as well as living more in harmony with the climate. The fruits help us adapt to seasonal changes in the summer and autumn. As summer progresses, the fruits become more abundant and sweeter – it puts us in touch with what's happening in the world around us. Look to the food lists at the end of this chapter.

SOY FOODS – GIFTS FROM THE EAST

Soy foods are rapidly gaining popularity as an alternative to both meat and dairy. Soy was recognized in many Asian countries as an excellent source of protein. Studies have shown that women who get their protein from soy are less likely to have problems with the menopause and may even have a lower rate of hormone-related cancers. This phenomenon is undoubtedly due to the fact that the soy bean contains nutrients that mimic the activity of certain human hormones. To gain the maximum benefit, a number of traditional ways of processing were discovered to make it tasty and easy to assimilate.

The product most familiar in the West is Tofu. Tofu is made by curdling soy milk which is then pressed into blocks. It has a fairly neutral taste and takes on the taste of other foods it is combined with. It can be used in soups, vegetable dishes and even used in desserts. It comes in various consistencies: soft, medium and hard. It is also used in some prepared foods such as sausages, meat substitutes and cheese substitutes. Dried tofu is also available and tasty in vegetable dishes. The nutritional concentration in dried tofu makes it an excellent health food. Use only the light brown coloured product; the white ones have been dyed. Try and use the organic and non-GMO varieties.

Miso is a food developed in Japan by fermenting the soybean. The fermentation process can produce Tamari, Shoyu (naturally produced soy sauces) and Miso. Miso is a paste that can be used in much the same way we would use bouillon. It can be used in making sauces, soups and snack foods. The natural soy sauces are used primarily as a cooking condiment. Miso is especially good for general health and is known as a healing food in Japan. The fermentation process breaks down the nutrients, making them very available to the body – it is the most nutritionally concentrated way of using soy. It is a naturally fermented product that is beneficial to intestinal flora. There are several types of miso, each with a different flavour; experiment and find out which ones you prefer. Stay with naturally produced and preferably organic products.

Tempeh, which originates in Indonesia, is now readily available in health shops. It comes in pressed cakes and can be cut to size for use in any number of recipes. It has a meaty taste and can be used as a substitute for meat in any dish.

Soymilk is now available in most supermarkets and can be used in place of milk; try to avoid those brands that have added sugar.

SEASONAL EATING

The issue of environment can, and should, come into play with food choices. Even though most of us don't work outside (or even go outside, except to walk to the car), the seasons still change and our bodies know it. Having big juicy steaks in the summer and ice cream in the winter doesn't make any sense. Our body knows what season it is and we need to respect its needs. In the summer we want to cool down and be more active; in the winter we need to keep warm and are more laid back (that doesn't mean not exercising).

In Asian medicine the concept of seasonal eating was very important. If we were simply living off the land, this wouldn't be a problem. What we need in each season is what grows – pretty neat, I'd say. Most of us would be really bored through, me included. Even though modern transportation and refrigeration gives us a huge variety of foods in all seasons, keeping track of what your body needs is a good idea. If you can nudge your diet to a more sensible seasonal rhythm, you will notice a difference. When you pay attention to the seasons you will notice that you have fewer colds and a greater resistance to ill health. In the chart below we can see the cycle of energy in the plant-growing cycle.

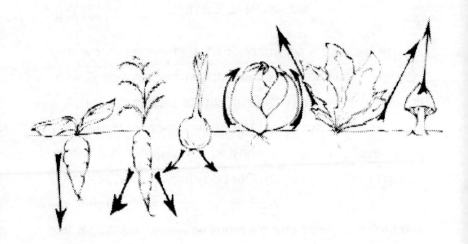

A THEME FOR EVERY SEASON

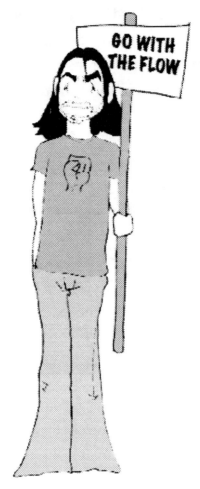

WINTER is when the vegetal energy is at its lowest ebb. This is the time when we need to warm up. Nature demonstrates to us that winter is a time of hibernation and stillness. Growth ceases as nature rests. The body thickens; we often gain a few pounds in preparation for the period of hibernation. We require this extra body fat to keep our kidneys warm during the long cold months. Using more oil in cooking, stews and hearty soups with beans and root vegetables can really provide lasting warmth. This is a good time of year for softer grain dishes and porridges in the morning, food that "sticks to your ribs".

If you use fish, fowl or meat, cook it in stews or serve with plenty of vegetables. Even a better option is using dried tofu or tempeh in those stews and thick soups. All the root vegetables are of real value in the winter – use carrots, turnips, as well as cabbage and kale. Kasha (buckwheat) is a great grain to try in the winter; it has been used for centuries in cold climates to generate heat. Sea vegetables will be used in the recipes in the next chapter; they are especially good in the winter stews and are amazing sources of trace minerals.

SPRING is a time when the heavier eating of the winter needs a clean up. We clean our houses in the spring, why not our bodies? Winter food has a tendency to be more fatty and have more protein. Foods like bean sprouts, raw foods and a concentration on vegetables as opposed to meat or fish. As the weather turns sunny, this is a good time to get into the outdoors and hike, walk and play.

Now is a good time to cut down a little on food volume. Cleansing foods like vinegar in salad dressings or in cooking, radish or spring onions used as a garnish, should be used along with ginger or lemon. Endive and beetroot are good choices as well as using a lighter grain such as barley or bulgur wheat.

SUMMER is the time of greatest expansion of energy in the cycle. It is the most abundant time for growth. The foods that are most needed when the weather is warm are salads, fruits, green vegetables and lighter cooking. Cooking needs to be subtle as well, not overcooking. This kind of food will help us keep our cool. If we use animal food in our diet, the amount used needs to be reduced or, better yet, eliminated.

This is the best time of year to lose weight, so choose foods which are simple, eat salads and fresh fruits – the whole diet should be of a cooler, lighter nature. Keep the heat outside and do less cooking. Seasonal foods such as cress, varieties of lettuce, tomato and spinach are very helpful.

It is good to resist the habit of drinking cold beverages. These cool you off for a short period of time and then you get hot again. If you do drink them, take it slower and you will find you are more comfortable. Use soft fruits and berries to cool down. Introduce cous-cous, bulgur wheat or quinoa into your salads and add fresh corn to your diet.

LATE SUMMER is a season of its own in Chinese medicine. It is that time when the first hints of autumn are present but the leaves have not yet fallen. It is a time when "sweet cooking" is recommended. This means that there is more roasting of vegetables so that they caramelize and the sugars are released. The grains for this season are millet and rice. Late fruits such as pears and apples are fresh and good in desserts. White bean dishes and Garbanzo beans (chick peas) are good choices.

AUTUMN is a time when energy starts to descend in the vegetable kingdom. It is a season of change as winter approaches; there is often a fluctuation between cool and warm days. Root vegetables, squash, cabbage, hearty greens like broccoli and kale, more grain and bean dishes and slightly longer cooking times are good in the fall. This is a good time to start some winter cooking – hearty soups and rice dishes. Miso soups are especially good. This is a good time to perk up the lungs before the cold weather hits.

Onions, garlic, chives and leeks (all part of the *allium* group) are good to treat chest complaints and help keep the airways open and clear. Garlic and peppers (remember those antioxidants) could be considered as agents to strengthen the immune system.

WHAT TO EAT

What is listed below is pretty close to the foods listed in the Macrobiotic diet. I do not follow the diet strictly (where would the *Pino Grigio* go?) but it is the best guideline I know of. In fact, many people have taken freely from it and not given credit where credit is due. You can use this as a starting point for getting your diet in line. If you have specific nutritional requirements or allergies, you should consult a professional.

Whole Cereal Grains are the foundation; year round they should comprise from 30% to 50% of the volume of food eaten daily. Use more grain in the winter and less in the summer. When losing weight, use less. Cooked whole grains are preferable to flour products, as they are more nutritionally complete. Whole cereal grains and wholegrain products include: short-grain brown rice, medium-grain brown rice, millet, barley, corn, whole oats, wheat groats, rye, buckwheat and quinoa. These grains are the ones that are used most often. Grains and grain products, which have less nutritional punch are: long-grain brown rice, basmati rice, wholewheat noodles, udon noodles, soba noodles, un-yeasted wholewheat bread, rye bread, rice cakes, cracked wheat, bulgur, steel-cut oats, rolled oats, corn grits, cornmeal, rye flakes, couscous.

Fresh vegetables prepared in a variety of ways, including steaming, boiling, baking, pressure cooking or sautéing (with a small amount of sesame, corn, or other vegetable oil) should comprise from 25% to 40% of daily food consumption by volume.

Green and White Leafy Vegetables for regular use include: pak choi, carrot tops, Chinese cabbage, collard greens, daikon greens, dandelion greens, kale, mustard greens, parsley, scallion, turnip greens, watercress, leeks, celery, cucumber, endive, romaine lettuce, rocket, sprouts, mangetout, peas.

Stem/Root Vegetables for regular use include: carrots, turnip, yam, onion, swede, parsnip, daikon (long white radish).

Note: the potato is not really a nutritional winner; use them as a comfort food but stick to the others for nutritional punch. They don't combine well with whole grains either.

Ground Vegetables for regular use include: cauliflower, cabbage, broccoli, Brussels sprouts, winter squash, butternut squash, pumpkin, red cabbage, summer squash and courgette.

A small portion of 10% to 15% of daily meals should include cooked beans or soy products. This may include: aduki beans, black-eye peas, chickpeas (garbanzos), kidney beans, split peas, lentils (green), white beans, pinto beans, soybeans, dried peas, broad beans, fava beans or a serving of tofu or tempeh.

Note: fish or other animal proteins do not combine well with beans.One or two bowls of soup seasoned with miso or tamari-soy sauce is a good idea everyday. The flavour should be mild, not too salty and not too bland. Prepare soups with a variety of ingredients, changing them daily. Include a variety of seasonal vegetables, sea vegetables, especially wakame or kombu, and occasionally add grains and/or beans.

Sea Vegetables can be an important addition to your diet. There are a variety of options and each has its special uses. Just a few small portions a week and you will be getting an amazing spectrum of trace minerals. Sea vegetables are prepared in a variety of ways, for example in soup, with beans (kombu is especially recommended) or as side dishes. Sea vegetable dishes may be flavoured with a moderate amount of tamari-soy sauce and brown rice vinegar. Sea vegetables for regular use include: kombu, (for soup stocks, as a side dish or condiment), wakame (in soups, especially miso soup, or in salad), nori (as a garnish) hijiki or arame (as a side dish), or dulse (in soups or salads).

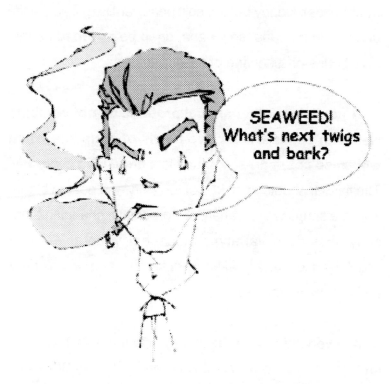

Nuts and seeds can be used daily as a garnish or a snack. Pumpkin seeds, sesame seeds, sunflower seeds, flax seeds, almonds, walnuts, hazelnuts and cashews can be eaten raw or roasted lightly.

If you eat fish or any other animal food, it is best eaten with a good portion of vegetables and partially refined grain rather than wholegrain.

Using bulgur, couscous, refined rice or pastas make for better complement.

Desserts are best when sweetened with a high quality sweetener, especially those made from grains. Only locally grown fruits are recommended. If you live in a temperate zone, try to limit the use of tropical or semi-tropical fruit. Some natural sweeteners are rice syrup, barley malt, dried raisins or fruit juices. Among the temperate climate fruits are: apples, strawberries, cherries, blueberries, watermelon, cantaloupe, Peaches, Plums, Raspberries, Pears, Apricots, and Grapes.

Note: it is best to eat fruit at least one hour after having a meal with significant amounts of whole grain.

Pure water is the best drink. In the environment chapter we will talk about water quality and the amazing Pi water technology. We all need between six and eight glasses a day, that's good quality pure water, every day. There are a wide variety of herbal teas available now. Green tea and bancha tea are noted for their rich content of antioxidants.

Note: alcoholic beverages actually dehydrate you, so does coffee, commercial teas and fizzy drinks – what a deal!

Use only high quality, cold-pressed vegetable oil. Good oil should be stored in a cool dark place and used in moderation. Its primary use should be for sautéing vegetables. When you are heating the oil to a high temperature, use olive oil or sesame oil – they do not lose their nutrient value as easily in high heat.

Seasonings are supposed to be way in the background. Let the food speak for itself. As you simplify your diet you will notice that you become more sensitive to the tastes in your food. It's a lovely surprise bonus to getting healthy.

Naturally processed, unrefined sea salt is preferable over other varieties.

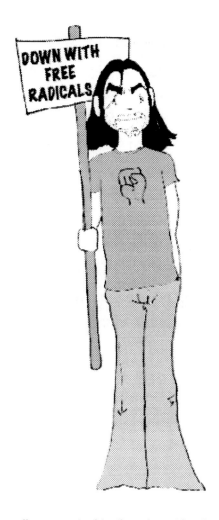

If we are all connected to the planet by the life force, then what we do has an effect on the planet as well as the other way around. We know that we affect the environment by our choices but sometimes we view this as something abstract. Food is a good example of how natural justice works. (Natural justice is simply the way that energy creates balance.)

Life force wants to create balance in all living things. Food is one of the most important exchanges of energy on the planet. When we abuse the abundance of food available, imbalances occur. In the industrial countries of the world we consume more food than is needed to live a healthy life. We also depend on animal farming to form the basis of our eating habits.

Animal farming is wasteful as a primary form of food. We feed grains and beans to animals and cut down forests to create grazing land. The grains fed to animals are wasted. There is only one pound of protein-rich food produced for every five pounds we feed to the animal. In the 70s an American woman called Francis Lappe-Moore wrote a wonderful book called *Diet for a Small Planet* about this terrible situation; it is worth a read. This creates an energy imbalance. We are taking more than we need. People are starving in the world when there is enough food to go around if we would change our ways.

The result in the richer nations is that the imbalance makes us sick, really sick. Up to 50% of all degenerative illness is due to poor diet. Cancer, heart disease, diabetes and obesity: these diseases are all due to the fact that we refuse to see the planet as a whole. Don't mess with the life force.

Eating a good diet should be good for everyone. A good diet should be a diet that can feed the world, that's cheap, that supports the soil, which respects life. If we all started to work in that direction it would be wonderful – just little steps can make a difference.

Stella – Burning Brighter Every Day

Dear Marlene

Happiness comes when work and words are of benefit to you and others.

This is so true for me as over a year ago I was introduced to you and the Academy of Wellness. Overweight, and I thought, living a comfortable life. However, something was not quite right. Comfortable is not good. Exciting and challenging is.

Marlene with your focus on life determination, knowledge, passion and compassion you listened and you taught me about my body and my mind.

My body is now 2 stones lighter, well toned, and all my internal organs (old but still functioning) are being exercised and I now realise that they were my responsibility. I now nourish them with good nutrition, (healthy eating), drinking water (remember the water Stella) and my Personal Training with you. You even convinced me to drink green tea!

You gave me back my confidence and energy, which made me realise that my dreams and aspirations can be fulfilled and not snuffed out like a candle.

Everyone has something to offer and nobody has the right to pull that magic carpet from under you.

Marlene you have taught me to realise that yesterday's inhibitions are history, learn from the past and move on. There is a big wide world out there with room for everyone. My attitude has changed to more of a positive nature and I feel fantastic.

Thank you for everything.

Love Stella

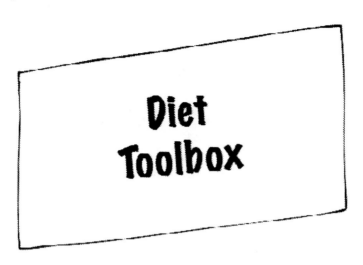

Diet Toolbox

This is a very long chapter with a very short toolbox. Here are just a few reminders for you to think about.

Eat low down on the food chain. There's nothing you can't get with a diet that is vegetarian. If you are going to eat meat, eat lean, and shop for meat that is not raised with hormones. Prefer fowl to beef, pork or lamb, prefer fish to fowl, prefer bean products to all of them.

Read labels, read labels, read labels. The more ingredients, the less you want it. If an ingredient has more than three syllables, it was probably produced by a chemist, not Mother Nature.

Don't eat before going to bed. Eating is for energy – you need very little energy to sleep. When we eat before sleeping the body is trying to digest food rather than getting down into deep sleep. The food we have eaten is often not digested properly and contributes to acid reflux and a variety of problems with the digestive system.

Sit down and slow down when you eat. Give the food a chance. Food needs respect, it needs attention, it needs digestion. When we eat on the run we diminish the nutritional value of the food. Slow down and pay attention.

Junk food is just that – don't eat it and don't give it to the kids. Educating kids doesn't mean creating a prison camp where they only eat porridge. Find out the kind of foods the kids like and do your best to meet them part way. When they are out of sight they will eat what they want anyway. Just set down reasonable guidelines for the home. You do control what they eat at home – make it the best food possible.

Don't starve yourself, enjoy your food and eat till you are full. If you are eating good food and exercising regularly, don't worry so much about volume. If you are really overdoing it and you know it, try chewing. Most of us will bolt our food down as if there were a race, if left to our own accord. Best way to make sure you chew well is to put down the utensils after you put food in your mouth. It may seem ridiculous at first but when you have spoon or fork in hand you are ready to fill up again. Set them down and chew till your food is approaching liquid.

Eat organically as much as possible. It is important that we support those people who care enough about the land to care for it. Organic farming not only saves the soil but also produces food with a higher nutritional value and a better taste. Why have a dose of chemical pesticides and herbicides with dinner?

Supplements are sometimes a good idea. I am not a big believer in taking a lot of pills, but the quality of our food has gone down a lot in past years. This fact along with increased environmental challenge leads me to use some supplementation. I use a concentrated barley enzyme and an antioxidant. I have felt the difference and will talk about these in the last chapter.

Buy a blender. You will find that making fruit smoothies and other fruit desserts with a blender saves time and is a blessing on a busy day.

If you slip off the path don't fall off the cliff.
Choosing a healthy life is about enjoying life
and having fun. If you slip off your diet plan,
don't get depressed – review how it happened
and get refocused. Don't make yourself crazy
and don't make other people crazy (that's my
job). Have fun.

CHAPTER SIX
RECIPES FOR HEALTHY LIVING

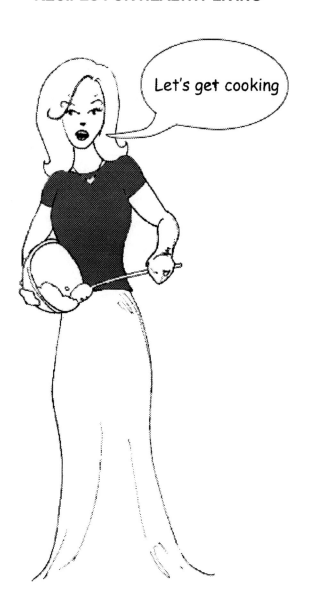

Here are a few of my favourite soups, salads, and other delicious and easy to make dishes. I cannot over emphasise how important it is to use fresh produce. Fresh food gives you the most concentrated range of vitamins, minerals, fibre and antioxidants. These are ingredients we all need for good health and slowing down the aging process.

I have, according everyone who comes through my kitchen, the 'biggest' soup pot they have ever seen! Why? Because if I only had a small soup pot I would only make small quantities of soup, so when I am hungry and I have been training with clients throughout the day I will keep my energy levels topped up with whatever delicious soup is in my BIG soup pot. There is always a pot of soup at the ready and it's a great 'habit'.

Having seeds and nuts to use as a condiment is a good idea. They can be added to salads or your morning porridge. I keep an airtight container in my kitchen cupboard with my own mixture. I mix in high fibre bran, wheat germ, sesame seeds, linseed, pumpkin seeds, and almonds, delicious.

OATS

Oats are one of the most nutritious grains. Oatmeal and rolled oats go through minimal processing, so they are whole foods, losing little of their nutritional properties.

Oats are full of protein and minerals and are helpful for building bones, teeth and connective tissue and for boosting energy generally. They also contain high levels of calcium and phosphorous and are easily digested. Their soluble fibre content acts on the digestive system in several ways. They provide dietary bulk, which improves the digestive process and help prevent constipation. They sweep food – and carcinogens through the gut and that may also help prevent bowel cancer.

One of the most significant benefits is in helping to maintain cardiovascular health. Their soluble fibre helps to lower cholesterol and generally boost cardiovascular health, lowering high blood pressure. In the colder months in particular it is a fantastic way to get your body moving. A bowl of porridge being the best know cooked recipe will set you up for the day.

All of my clients have taken this on board and they feel the benefits. Instead of rushing out the door in the morning without breakfast, be kind to your body. Remember, our bodies do not let us down we let our bodies down. Be innovative and add some tamari (soy sauce) or a drop of honey, depending on your preference to salt or sweet tasting porridge. Sprinkle some sesame seeds, or pumpkin seeds, wheat germ or bran on top for a healthy nutritious breakfast. Generations of Scots can't be wrong!

CEREAL GRAINS
Short-grain Brown Rice with Squash

This is a delicious dish and when the squash is so sweet you would swear it was sugared if you didn't know better.

2 cups short-grain brown rice, rinsed
1 cup cubed winter squash
3 cups spring or filtered water
2 pinches sea salt
1 tablespoon barley miso
slivered nori sheets or minced parsley, for garnish

Combine rice, squash and water in a pressure cooker and cook over medium heat, uncovered, until the mixture comes to a boil. Add salt. Seal and bring to full pressure. Place over a flame deflector, reduce heat to low and cook for 50 minutes.

Meanwhile, purée miso in a small amount of water and simmer it for 3–4 minutes. When the rice is cooked, remove it from heat and allow pressure to reduce naturally. Stir puréed miso into hot rice and transfer to a serving bowl. Serve garnished with nori seaweed or parsley.

Short-grain Brown Rice

Buy some short-grain brown rice and if you have a pressure cooker, cook half a pack in a small amount of water – this will give you enough brown rice for a good few days.

Make various additions to it by sautéing some onions, carrots, mushrooms, broccoli, or whatever your choice.

You can use the rice for a few days after you cook it and add it to stir-fries, soups or stews. If your kitchen is cool, you can leave it in a covered container; if not, put it in the fridge. If it thickens, heat it up with some water in the pot before adding it to your vegetables.

Fried Rice and Vegetables

This vegetarian recipe relies on an abundance of fresh vegetables and flavoured seasoning that creates a low-fat, delicious alternative to the oily and salty standard.

1–2 teaspoons dark sesame oil
3 or 4 slices ginger root, cut into thin matchsticks
sea salt
1/4 cup each sliced onion, carrot matchsticks, burdock matchsticks,
thinly sliced button mushrooms and shredded cabbage

1–2 cups cooked short-grain brown rice

1–2 stalks broccoli, broken into florets

soy sauce

brown rice vinegar

parsley sprigs, for garnish

Heat oil in a skillet. Add ginger root and a pinch of salt and cook, stirring, until golden. Add onion and another pinch of salt and cook, stirring, until onion is translucent – about 5 minutes. Add carrot, burdock, mushrooms and another pinch of salt and cook, stirring occasionally, until coated with oil. Finally, stir in cabbage and another pinch of salt and cook until cabbage begins to wilt – about 5 minutes.

Spread vegetables evenly over the skillet and top with cooked rice, then broccoli. Sprinkle lightly with soy sauce. Gently add about 1/8 inch of water to allow everything to steam together, cover and cook over medium heat for about 10 minutes, until all liquid is absorbed and broccoli is cooked. Turn off heat and season to taste with rice vinegar. Stir well, transfer to a serving bowl and garnish with parsley sprigs.

Millet

Millet is a short cooking grain. Two parts of water to one part of millet, bring to a boil, then turn down and simmer till cooked. Keep a flame spreader or make sure that the flame is not too high or the millet will burn.

If you roast the millet in a slightly oiled pan before cooking, it brings out a lovely nutty taste. Just oil the pan, heat and add the millet. Keep the millet moving with a wooden spoon till some of the grains begin to pop; remove and cook.

Brown Rice and Millet Croquettes

With some imagination you can be creative with grain.

1/2 cup cooked brown rice
1/2 cup cooked millet
1/4 cup combined diced onion and carrot
1/4 cup fresh corn kernels (optional)
fine yellow or white cornmeal
safflower oil for deep frying or shallow frying

Combine grains and vegetables in a large bowl. With moist hands, form the croquettes into small rounds, thick discs or oblong fingers. Pour some cornmeal onto a plate and gently pat croquette until completely coated.

This will hold the croquette together as well as give it a crispy coating.

To deep-fry, heat about 1 inch of oil in a heavy skillet or pan over medium heat. Deep-fry each croquette until golden brown. Drain well on paper towels to remove excess oil. If shallow frying, heat about 1/4 inch of oil in a skillet over medium heat. Fry the croquettes on each side until golden. Drain well on paper towels.

You can serve these with Creamy Sesame Dressing or a Garlic, Mushroom and Leek Sauce or a simple dipping sauce consisting of soy sauce, water and fresh ginger juice or lemon juice.

Nutty Rice and Broccoli

2 cups brown rice, rinsed

2.5 cups spring or filtered water

2 pinches sea salt

2 cups broccoli florets

1/4 cup diced carrot

1/4 cup diced red onion

1/2 cup walnut pieces

1 teaspoon barley miso, dissolved in a little water

grated peel of 1 lemon

Combine rice and water in a pressure cooker. Bring to a boil, loosely covered, over medium heat. Add salt, seal and bring to full pressure. Place over a flame deflector, reduce heat to low and cook for 45 minutes. Remove from heat and allow pressure to reduce naturally.

While the rice is cooking, bring a pan of water to a boil. Separately, cook broccoli, carrot and onion in boiling water until crisp-tender, cool in cold water and drain. Mix vegetables together in a medium bowl. Set aside.

Heat a dry skillet over medium heat. Add the walnuts and pan-toast until fragrant, about 5 minutes, stirring. Purée walnuts and miso until a coarse paste forms. Stir vegetables, walnut paste and lemon peel into rice. Transfer to a serving bowl.

Brown Rice Risotto

1.5 cups medium-grain brown rice
2 teaspoons light sesame oil
1/4 cup mirin
3/4 cup spring or filtered water
5 cups vegetable stock
1/4 cup leek, rinsed well and thinly sliced
1/2 cup diced carrot

Soak rice in water to cover 6–8 hours. Drain and discard the soaking water. Heat 1 teaspoon of the oil in a deep skillet over medium heat. Add rice and a pinch of salt and cook, stirring, until coated with oil. Stir in mirin and water, cover and cook, stirring frequently, over medium heat. As soon as rice absorbs the liquid, begin adding vegetable stock in ? cup amounts, stirring frequently, but cook rice covered instead of the traditional method of cooking risotto in an uncovered pan. As rice absorbs liquid, continue adding stock until all the stock has been used, 40–45 minutes. Taste the rice to be sure that it is tender before removing from heat.

Heat the remaining oil in a skillet over medium heat. Add leeks and a pinch of salt and cook, stirring, until limp. Add carrots and a pinch of salt and cook until tender. Stir vegetables into the risotto and serve warm.

Bulgur with Skillet Veggies

You can serve this with a fresh salad or a light soup.

1–2 tablespoons light sesame oil

1 onion diced

1 clove garlic, minced

sea salt

1 cup bulgur wheat

2 cups spring or filtered water

2 cups thinly sliced fresh button mushrooms,

brushed clean

1 cup small cauliflower florets

1 carrot, cut into thin matchsticks

7 or 8 Brussels sprouts, halved and thinly sliced

soy sauce

generous pinch of dried rosemary

1 tablespoon kuzu, dissolved in a little cold water

2 tablespoons slivered almonds, pan-toasted

Heat sesame oil in a skillet over medium heat. Add onion, garlic and a pinch of sea salt and sauté until translucent, 2–3 minutes. Add bulgur and cook, stirring constantly, about 2 minutes. Gently add water and a pinch of salt and bring to a boil. Cover, reduce heat and cook 15 minutes, until liquid is absorbed.

In another skillet over medium heat, arrange mushrooms, cauliflower, carrot and Brussels sprouts around the skillet, each in its own section. Add enough water to half cover, sprinkle lightly with soy sauce and bring to a boil. Cover, reduce heat and simmer until cauliflower is crisp-tender, about 6 minutes. Add rosemary to taste and stir in dissolved kuzu. Cook, stirring, until liquid is slightly thickened. Transfer bulgur to a serving bowl and top individual servings with vegetables and almonds.

Oriental-style Millet

1 cup millet, rinsed

3 cups spring or filtered water

soy sauce

1–2 teaspoons dark sesame oil

3–4 slices ginger root, minced

2 cloves garlic, minced

1 small carrot, finely diced

1 onion, cut into thin diagonal slices

1 teaspoon fresh ginger juice

1 teaspoon brown rice syrup

1 tablespoon brown rice vinegar

2 tablespoons shelled peanuts, pan-toasted

Heat a deep, dry skillet over medium heat. Drain millet well before toasting so that it toasts evenly and doesn't burn. Add to skillet and toast for about 5 minutes, until millet puffs and begins to pop. Add water and a sprinkle of soy sauce and bring to a boil. Reduce heat, cover and simmer for 30 minutes or until the liquid is nearly absorbed. Remove from heat and allow to stand, covered, 10 minutes. Fluff with a fork and transfer to a serving bowl.

Heat sesame oil in a skillet over medium heat. Add ginger and garlic, cook 2–3 minutes. Add carrot and onions and cook until tender, 2–3 minutes. Sprinkle with a little soy sauce and stir in ginger juice and rice syrup. Remove from heat and stir in rice vinegar and peanuts. Fold into hot millet. Serve warm, as millet tends to stiffen as it cools.

Quinoa with Tempeh and Parsley

Quinoa cooks up very quickly – you could call it healthy "fast food".

1 cup quinoa

2 cups spring or filtered water

pinch of sea salt

safflower oil for deep-frying

1 x 8 oz pack of tempeh, cubed

1 teaspoon, extra-virgin olive oil

1 clove garlic, minced

1 onions, cut into thin diagonal slices

soy sauce

2 celery stalks, diced

juice of 1 lime

1/4 cup parsley, chopped fine

Place quinoa in a fine strainer and rinse well. This is especially important because the grains are covered with a coating of a substance called saponin, which protects the delicate grains. If not rinsed off, this substance can make your cooked grain taste bitter. Place in a pot with water and bring to the boil. Add salt. Cover, reduce heat and simmer about 30 minutes until liquid is absorbed and quinoa is fluffy. Set aside.

Heat about 1 inch of safflower oil in a heavy skillet or pan over medium heat. Test the oil temperature by dropping in a piece of tempeh. If it sinks and comes immediately back to the top, the oil is hot enough to deep-fry properly. (Remember the point of deep-frying) is to add richness to your diet and to give you the strong kind of energy present only in cooking foods over high heat, very quickly. Deep-fry the tempeh cubes until golden brown. Drain on paper towels and set aside.

Heat the olive oil in a skillet over medium heat. Add the garlic, onions and a little soy sauce and cook until onions are tender, about 3 minutes. Stir in celery, quinoa and tempeh and toss well. Remove from heat and stir in lime juice and parsley. Serve warm.

Carrot and Sweet Potato Pilaf

This rice dish is enlivened by the sweetness of carrots and sweet potato.

1 tbsp olive oil

1 onion, peeled and sliced

1 medium sweet potato, peeled and cubed

4 carrots, peeled and chopped

250 g (9 oz) brown basmati rice

500 ml (16 fl oz) vegetable stock (bouillon)

125 g (4 oz) dried apricots, halved

small bunch parsley and mint, chopped

50 g (2 oz) pine nuts, toasted

In a large, heavy-based pan, heat the oil and add onion, sweet potato and carrots, and fry over a fairly high heat until onion is softened and vegetables are starting to colour.

Stir in rice, then pour in stock and dried apricots. Season with sea salt and freshly ground black pepper if preferred. Cover and bubble for about 10–15 minutes, until rice is cooked and vegetables are tender.

Remove from heat and stir in herbs and pine nuts before serving.

SEA VEGETABLES

Sea vegetables are some of the best available sources of a whole range of important minerals, including calcium, iron, potassium, zinc, silicon and iodine.

When clients tell me they are on thyroxine medication to help alleviate the symptoms of an under-active thyroid, I always advise them to start incorporating seaweeds into their diet, as they truly are mineral treasures from the depth of the sea. Iodine is needed for the thyroid gland to function properly; without it the body's metabolism slows down, becoming prone to goitre. Seaweed contains even higher levels of iodine than fish. Seaweed is an effective detoxifier and is particularly valuable as increasing evidence shows that it reduces the risk of developing cancer.

I have listed a few seaweed recipes that I enjoy.

Stir-fried Arame Seaweed with Tofu

Arame is usually available in shredded form and can be steamed, sautéed or eaten cold. It can also be used in soups or salads. Arame seaweed has a firm texture, which contrasts with tofu. This is a simple stir-fry that can be assembled at the last minute once the tofu has been fried and the seaweed soaked. Serve hot with freshly boiled brown rice or leave to cool and serve as a chilled salad with grilled teriyaki salmon.

500 g (1lb) firm tofu
25–50 g (1–2 oz) rice flour or plain flour, for dusting
10–12 tablespoons groundnut oil, for frying
15 g (1/2 oz) arame seaweed
2 garlic cloves, crushed
3 tablespoons light soy sauce
6 tablespoons mirin
2 teaspoons clear honey
4 tablespoons sesame oil
2 spring onions or 6 mangetout, finely shredded
boiled brown rice, to serve

Cut the tofu into thick slices and dust them in rice flour or plain flour. Heat 8–10 tablespoons of the groundnut oil in a frying pan and fry the pieces of tofu, two at a time, for about 2–4 minutes, turning them once or until golden brown on all sides. Remove the tofu from the oil and drain on kitchen paper. Reserve the oil.

Soak the arame seaweed in boiling water for 30 minutes. Remove the seaweed and reserve the soaking water. Roughly chop any larger strands of seaweed. Strain the soaking water and put 6 tablespoons into a saucepan with the garlic, soy sauce, mirin and honey and heat gently for 5 minutes.

Heat the remaining 2 tablespoons of groundnut oil in a wok or large frying pan. Return the tofu to the oil with the seaweed and stir-fry for 1 minute. Add the mirin and soy mixture to the hot pan and stir-fry quickly. Add the sesame oil and shredded spring onions or mangetout and serve with boiled brown rice.

Seaweed and Cucumber Salad with Rice Wine Vinegar Dressing

Remember that seaweed is packed with iron, calcium and potassium. This salad is best made with the mixed bags of seaweed and sea lettuces available in Chinese and Oriental stores, or some local supermarkets are now stocking them. Is that not fantastic! We are definitely moving in the right direction. The world is changing, with more and more people looking for healthy food.

Serve this salad as a starter or snack with miso soup,   or as a side dish with grilled fish.

25 g (1 oz) mixed dried seaweed, such as dulse and sea lettuce
1 small cucumber
75 ml (3 fl oz) mirin
75 ml (3 fl oz) rice wine vinegar
2 tablespoons lemon juice

Place the seaweed in a bowl, cover with cold water and leave to stand for 15–20 minutes to soften.

Cut the cucumber in half lengthways, then slice it very thinly into half-moons. Drain the seaweed and roughly chop any large pieces. Put the chopped seaweed in a bowl with the sliced cucumber.

Mix the mirin with the rice wine vinegar and add the lemon juice.

Pour the dressing over the seaweed and cucumber and toss lightly. Serve in small mounds in individual bowls.

BEANS AND SOY PRODUCTS

This extensive and nutritious family of foods includes red, green and brown lentils, red, white and black kidney beans, chickpeas, and haricot, aduki, flageolet, black-eyed, mung and butter beans. The versatile soya bean is treated separately.

The most important part for me is the fact that the oestrogen connection with pulses becomes paramount, as I am now going through the menopause. As pulses contain phytoestrogens, or plant oestrogens, which occur naturally in certain plants and mimic female hormones, then these phytoestrogens have a stabilizing effect on the menstrual cycle; they are believed to be highly beneficial in regulating erratic periods, tackling PMS and relieving menopausal symptoms, such as hot flushes and night sweats. They are used increasingly as an alternative to HRT (hormone replacement therapy). There is also increasing evidence that pulses lower breast cancer risks and protect against fibroids, (benign tumours) in the uterus, most common in childless, pre-menopausal women over the age of 35, and they also have a steadying effect on blood sugar levels. The other interesting fact is that, since I started to take a daily dose of black cohosh, which contains 200mg of soya, my body is feeling more like ME again. I believe that many people avoid using beans etc. in their diet because pulses can bring an unwanted side effect – flatulence. Mixing them with parsley, fennel, ginger or cayenne pepper can alleviate this.

I hope this information helps and, if you are suffering from the **'change of life'**, please try to incorporate beans, lentils (pulses) into your diet – you will be delighted with the results.

Try these recipes. They are easy to make and taste delicious.

Black Bean and Tofu Sausage Stew

750 g (1 lb 10 oz) dried black beans

1 tbsp olive oil

2 onions, finely chopped

4 garlic cloves, finely chopped

2 litres (3.5 pints) water

800 g (1 lb 12 oz) canned plum tomatoes in juice

1 tbsp tomato purée

1 bay leaf

1/2 teaspoon ground cumin

1/4 teaspoon dried oregano

1/2 tsp chilli purée

700 g (1 lb 9 oz) tofu sausages

salt and pepper (if desired)

To garnish

2–3 ripe avocados

3–4 tbsp lime juice

3 tomatoes, skinned, deseeded and chopped

about 300 ml (10 fl oz) soured cream

1 bunch spring onions, finely chopped

1 large bunch fresh coriander leaves, chopped

Soak the beans overnight.

Drain the beans, put in a saucepan and add enough cold water to cover by 5 cm (2 inches). Bring to the boil and boil for 10 minutes. Drain and rinse well.

Heat the oil in a very large pot or flameproof casserole over a medium heat. Add the onions and cook for about 5 minutes, stirring frequently, until they start to colour. Add the garlic and continue cooking for 1 minute.

Add the water, tomatoes, tomato purée and drained beans. When the mixture begins to bubble, reduce the heat to low. Add the bay leaf, cumin, oregano and chilli purée and stir to mix well. Cover and simmer for 1–2 hours, stirring occasionally, until the beans are very tender. Meanwhile bake the tofu sausages in a preheated oven at 180°C/350°F/Gas Mark 4 for 15 minutes, turning 2 or 3 times for even browning. Drain, slice and add to the beans after they have been cooking for about 1 hour.

Peel and dice the avocados. Mix with the lime juice in a bowl and turn to coat. Put all the other garnishes on your list in pretty separate bowls.

When the beans are tender, taste the soup and adjust the seasoning. Ladle the stew into warm bowls.

This is a lovely meal to share with friends and, of course, you can serve some lovely crackers or warm brown seeded bread to accompany the stew and the garnishes.

Tempeh

This is a delicious recipe and, as you now know, tempeh is a fermented soya bean cake and is an excellent source of protein.

125 g (4 oz) new potatoes

2 carrots

125 g (4 oz) bean sprouts

125 g (4 oz) green beans

175 g (6 oz) tempeh

4 hard-boiled eggs

8 cherry tomatoes, halved

handful of coriander leaves

Peanut Sauce

125 g (4 oz) peanuts, roasted

1 small fresh red chilli

2 shallots, finely chopped

3 garlic cloves, crushed

3 tablespoons soy sauce

1 tablespoon lime juice

1 tablespoon groundnut oil

sea salt and pepper

First make the peanut sauce. Grind the peanuts in a food processor until they are quite fine, then add the red chilli, shallots, crushed garlic, soy sauce, lime juice and salt and pepper (if desired) and blend for 1–2 minutes or until smooth.

Heat the oil in a saucepan, add the peanut paste and cook for 5 minutes, stirring constantly. Add 8 tablespoons water and stir well. Reduce the heat, cover the pan and simmer very gently for 30 minutes, adding more water if the sauce begins to dry out.

Cook the potatoes in boiling water for 8–10 minutes or until tender. Roughly slice them and arrange on 4 plates. Scrub the carrots and cut into matchsticks, or grate roughly, then mix with the bean sprouts. Trim the beans, cover with boiling water and blanch for 1 minute. Drain well and refresh in cold water.

Heat a dry pan, add the tempeh and toast on all sides until lightly brown. Remove the tempeh from the pan and slice into cubes.

Arrange the drained green beans on the potatoes, then add the carrots and bean sprouts, hard-boiled eggs and cherry tomatoes. Drizzle the peanut sauce over the salad and top with the coriander leaves. Serve immediately.

Simmered Lentils with Roasted Leeks

4 leeks, halved lengthways

4 tomatoes, halved

2 tablespoons olive oil

sea salt and cracked black pepper

simmered lentils

2 teaspoons olive oil

2 cloves garlic, sliced

315 g (10 oz) du puy lentils

3.75 cups (30 fl oz) vegetable stock

1/2 cup shredded fresh flat-leaf parsley

3 tablespoons lemon juice

Preheat the oven to 180°C (350°F). Place the leeks, cut-side up, on a baking tray and top with the tomatoes, also cut-side up. Drizzle with olive oil and sprinkle with salt and pepper. Bake for 40 minutes or until the leeks and tomatoes are soft.

To make the simmered lentils, place the oil in a frying pan over a medium heat. Add the garlic and cook for 1 minute or until soft. Add the lentils and the stock and simmer, covered, for 35 minutes or until just tender.

To serve, place the leeks and tomatoes on serving plates. Stir the parsley, lemon juice and some salt and pepper (if desired) through the lentils. Spoon over the leeks and tomatoes and serve.

Teriyaki Tofu and Vegetable Stir-fry

Tofu is a nutritious, low-fat ingredient made from soya beans. Its mild flavour means that it is best marinated before cooking.

3 tbsp teriyaki sauce
1 tbsp hot water
250 g (9 oz) tofu, dried in kitchen towel and cut into cubes
1 tbsp groundnut or vegetable oil
splash of toasted sesame oil
350 g (12 oz) broccoli florets
175 g (6 oz) fine green beans, trimmed
3 spring onions, sliced on the diagonal
4 pak choi, sliced in half
2 garlic cloves, chopped
6 tbsp fresh apple juice
4 tsp soy sauce
fresh coriander leaves, to garnish

Put the teriyaki sauce and water in a shallow dish. Add the tofu and carefully turn it in the sauce until completely coated. Cover with cling film and marinate in the fridge for around one hour.

Preheat the oven to 200°C/400°F/Gas Mark 6. Put the tofu and marinade in a roasting tin and cook for 20 minutes, turning occasionally, until slightly crisp and golden on the outside.

Meanwhile, heat a frying pan or wok and add both the groundnut and sesame oils. Add the broccoli and green beans, then stir-fry, tossing the vegetables continuously for 5 minutes.

Add the spring onions, pak choi, garlic and ginger and stir-fry for another 1 minute. Pour in the apple juice and soy sauce and cook for 1–2 minutes, adding a little extra water if the stir-fry appears dry.

Divide the stir-fry between 4 shallow bowls and top with the tofu. Garnish with coriander just before serving.

Fried Tempeh

Tempeh is available in better natural food stores. It is a soy product that is naturally processed. Read the label. Some tempeh has different added ingredients, such as seaweed or seeds.

The tempeh usually comes in a flat square piece. You can cut the tempeh any way you wish for cooking. For frying, the easiest way is to lay it flat and cut slices of about a .25 inch thick. The thinner the slices, the harder it is to keep them together when they cook.

Heat a skillet with a light coating of vegetable oil. Place the tempeh slices in it and cook about 3–4 minutes on each side. When the tempeh is cooking you can splash a few drops of soy sauce on the upper side. The tempeh will be a golden brown when done.

When you serve tempeh, you can use a spicy, sweet and sour or savoury sauce if you wish.

Tofu – cut into cubes and use in your miso soup or stir-fry with some garlic and sauté with some onions and mushrooms. Either way is delicious.

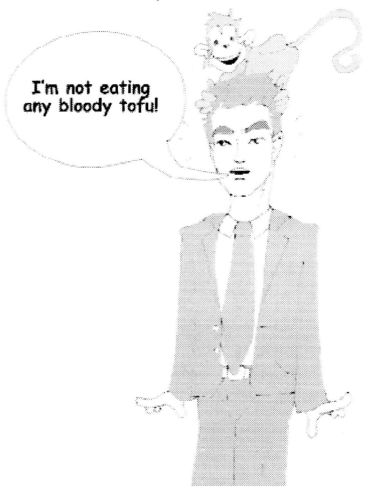

I'm not eating any bloody tofu!

Tofu Chow Mein

250 g ramen noodles

1 tbsp vegetable oil

3 spring onions, sliced

2 garlic cloves, finely chopped

2-cm piece fresh ginger root, peeled and finely chopped

285 g pack firm tofu, cut into small cubes

227 g can bamboo shoots, sliced

100 g (4 oz) bean sprouts

100 g (4 oz) mangetout, sliced lengthways

2 tbsp soy sauce

2 tbsp sweet chilli sauce

Cook the noodles according to the packet instructions. Meanwhile, heat the oil in a large frying pan or wok and stir-fry the spring onions, garlic and ginger for 1–2 minutes until slightly softened.

Add the tofu cubes and fry over a high heat for 2–3 minutes until golden. Stir in the bamboo shoots, bean sprouts and mangetout and stir-fry for a further 1–2 minutes.

Drain the noodles and add to the vegetables with the soy sauce and chilli sauce. Toss together and serve immediately.

SOUPS

Roasted Squash, Sweet Potato and Garlic Soup

1 large sweet potato
1 acorn squash
4 spring onions
olive oil
5–6 garlic cloves, unpeeled
850 ml (1.5 pints) stock (bouillon)
salt and pepper, if desired
snipped fresh chives, to garnish

Cut the sweet potato, squash and spring onions in half lengthways, through to the stem end. Brush the cut sides with oil.

Put the vegetables, cut-side down, in a shallow roasting tin. Add the garlic cloves. Roast in a preheated oven at 190°C/375°F/Gas Mark 5 for about 40 minutes until tender and light brown.

When cool, scoop the flesh from the sweet potato and squash halves and put in a saucepan with the spring onions. Remove the garlic peel and add the soft insides to the other vegetables.

Add the stock and bring to the boil, then reduce the heat and simmer, partially covered, for 30 minutes, stirring occasionally, until the vegetables are very tender.

Allow the soup to cool slightly then, using a hand blender, purée until smooth.

Ladle into warm bowls and garnish with snipped chives.

Miso Soup

Ingredients:

1	large onion
4	carrots
4	stalks of celery
3	6inch pieces of wakame seaweed
1	brick of tofu
3	tablespoons of miso paste

Wakame seaweed can be purchased at better health food store. It comes in a dried form.

Miso is a fermented soybean product that comes in a paste.

Cooking Instructions:

Break wakame into smaller pieces and soak in enough water to cover it. Wakame will soften in about 30min to an hour.

Sautee carrot, onion and celery in vegetable oil (sesame, canola, corn or olive) till lightly cooked.

Cut soft wakame into small pieces (quarter inch or so) and add to vegetables. Cover vegetables and wakame with 4 to 6 litres of water and bring to a boil. Turn heat down to a simmer and let cook for about one hour.

After the stock has cooked half an hour add the tofu (cut into small cubes)

Take approximately 3 tablespoons of miso paste and blend with half a cup of liquid from soup in a small bowel. Use a spoon to blend the miso and make sure it has dissolved. Add the miso to the soup. (You may want to add additional salt or miso or soy sauce to taste)

Serve hot and enjoy!

Vegetable Soup with Bulgur and Herbs

1 tbsp olive oil

2 onions, chopped

3 garlic cloves, finely chopped or crushed

50 g (1.75 oz) bulgur wheat

5 tomatoes, skinned and sliced

or 400 g (14 oz) canned plum tomatoes in juice

225 g (8 oz) peeled pumpkin or acorn squash, diced

1 large courgette, quartered lengthways and sliced

1 litre (1.75 pints) boiling water

2 tbs tomato purée

1/4 tsp chilli purée

40 g (1.5 oz) chopped mixed fresh oregano, basil and flat-leaf parsley

25 g (1 oz) rocket leaves, coarsely chopped

175 g (6 oz) shelled fresh or frozen peas

salt and pepper, if desired

freshly grated parmesan cheese, to serve

Heat the oil in a large saucepan over a medium-low heat and add the onions and garlic. Cover and cook for 5–8 minutes until the onions soften.

Stir in the bulgur wheat and continue cooking for 1 minute.

Layer the tomatoes, pumpkin and courgette in the saucepan.

Combine half the water with the tomato purée, chilli purée and a pinch of salt (optional). Pour over the vegetables. Cover and simmer for 15 minutes.

Uncover the saucepan and stir. Put all the herbs and the rocket on top of the soup and layer the peas over them. Pour over the remaining water and gently bring to the boil. Reduce the heat and simmer for about 20–25 minutes, or until all the vegetables are tender.

Stir the soup, taste and adjust the seasoning if required. Ladle into warm bowls and serve with parmesan cheese (if desired).

Spinach Soup

One of the most nutritious of the green, leafy vegetables, spinach is beneficial for a huge range of ailments, and protects and strengthens the body in numerous ways. It should not be eaten or drunk as a juice on a daily basis, however, as its cleansing effect can become too powerful. People with kidney or bladder stones should avoid it altogether because its oxalic acid content can exacerbate stones. There are many benefits to incorporating spinach into your diet, the main ones being lowering the risk of cancer; strengthening the immune system; preventing and relieving anaemia; constipation and normalizing high blood pressure.

1 tbsp olive oil
1 onion, halved and thinly sliced
1 leek split lengthways and thinly sliced
1 potato, finely diced
1 litre (1.75 pints) water
2 sprigs fresh marjoram or 1/4 tsp dried
2 sprigs fresh thyme or 1/4 tsp dried
1 bay leaf
400 g (14 oz) young spinach, washed
freshly grated nutmeg
salt and pepper, if required

Heat the oil in a heavy-based saucepan over a medium heat. Add the onion and leek and cook for about 3 minutes, stirring occasionally, until they begin to soften.

Add the potato, water, marjoram, thyme and bay leaf, along with a large pinch of salt (if you must!). Bring to the boil, reduce the heat, cover and cook gently for about 25 minutes until the vegetables are tender. Remove the bay leaf and the herb sprigs.

Add the spinach and continue cooking for 3–4 minutes, stirring frequently, just until it is completely wilted.

Allow the soup to cool slightly then, using a hand blender, purée the soup until smooth.

Add a generous serving of grated nutmeg and simmer for a few minutes. Ladle the soup into warm bowls and, if you so desire, swirl a tablespoon of cream into each serving.

Carrot and Red Lentil Soup

This thick nutritious soup is a good source of vitamins, minerals and fibre. Serve with seeded wholemeal rolls as a light meal.

The humble carrot is one of the great detoxifying foods. It not only cleanses, but it also regulates imbalances in the body. They work best when eaten raw as they release their natural sugars slowly into the body to give sustained energy, rather than the sudden burst that you get from refined sugars. Go on, start munching your way through a few carrot batons and promote healthy blood cells, heart and circulation – and they are great for the complexion.

1.5 tablespoons olive oil
1 large onion, chopped
1 celery stick, chopped
4 carrots, chopped
200 g (7 oz) red lentils, rinsed
2 fresh rosemary sprigs, each about 10 cm (4 inches) in length
1 bay leaf
1.4 litres (2.5 pints) vegetable stock
salt and pepper if desired

Heat the oil in a large heavy-based saucepan. Add the onion, cover the pan and cook for 8 minutes over a medium-low heat until softened. Add the celery and carrots, then cook for a further 3 minutes, stirring occasionally.

Add the lentils, rosemary, bay leaf and stock, then bring to the boil. Reduce the heat and simmer, half-covered, for 30 minutes or until the lentils are very soft. Occasionally skim off any foam that rises to the surface while cooking the lentils.

Remove the rosemary sprigs and bay leaf, then using a hand blender, blend the soup until smooth.

Ladle into warm bowls and season as required.

FISH

Fresh Tuna Niçoise

This main course salad is always a winner.

280 g (10 oz) small new potatoes, scrubbed

175 g (6 oz) fine green beans, trimmed

200 g (7 oz) cos lettuce, leaves separated and torn
into bite-sized pieces

50 g (1.5 oz) watercress

1 small red onion, thinly sliced

12 cherry tomatoes, halved

85 g (3 oz) black olives

olive oil, for brushing

juice of 1/2 lemon

4 tuna steaks, about 115 g (4 oz) each

1 tbsp chopped fresh flat-leaf parsley

salt and pepper, if desired

Dressing

1 tbsp extra-virgin olive oil

1 tsp white wine vinegar

3 tbsp mayonnaise

1 small garlic clove, crushed

Steam the potatoes and green beans until tender, using
separate saucepans. Drain the potatoes and leave to cool.

Refresh the green beans under cold running water and leave to cool.

Put the potatoes and green beans in a large serving bowl with the salad leaves, onion, tomatoes and olives.

Blend together the ingredients for the dressing and spoon it over the salad. Season as desired with salt and pepper and toss the salad with your hands until all the ingredients are coated.

Brush a griddle pan with some olive oil and heat until very hot. Squeeze the lemon juice over the tuna and season, then cook the fish for 4–5 minutes, turning once, until golden outside but slightly pink in the centre. Sprinkle with parsley and season if desired. Serve immediately with the salad.

Really Good Fish

You can serve this on a bed of millet, quinoa, rice or noodles for a delicious meal.

2 cloves garlic
small bunch of flat-leaf parsley
juice and zest of 1 lemon
juice and zest of 1 lime
4 salmon steaks, skin on
2 tbsp oil
2 red onions, sliced in wedges

150 ml (5 fl oz) vegetable stock

parsley, to garnish

In a food processor, add garlic, parsley, lemon and lime zest, and lime juice, with a good pinch of ground black pepper. Blitz to make a paste, taste and add sea salt if needed. Now spread it evenly over the top of the salmon steaks.

In a large frying pan, heat the oil and add the salmon, skin-side down. Cook for 2–3 minutes on each side, then remove from the pan and set aside. Add the spinach to the pan and fry for a few minutes until starting to shrink.

Throw in the onion and cook until softened. Now pour in the stock and lemon juice and bring to the boil. Place the fish steaks back in the pan, cover with a lid or foil and leave to steam for 2–3 minutes.

Sprinkle with some torn parsley and serve.

Leave the salmon's skin on while cooking, so the fish holds together – you can remove it before serving.

Haddock with a Twist

The tomato and herb salsa adds plenty of oomph to the simply cooked plain fish. Serve with steamed asparagus and broccoli.

4 thick haddock or cod fillets, about 200 g (7 oz) each

olive oil, for brushing

8 thin slices of lemon

salt and pepper

Salsa

8 vine-ripened tomatoes, deseeded and diced

2 shallots, diced

2 tbsp olive oil

1 garlic clove, crushed

3 tbsp chopped fresh parsley

3 tbsp chopped fresh basil

juice of 1 lemon

Preheat the oven to 200°C/400°F/Gas Mark 6. Rinse and dry each haddock fillet and place on a piece of foil that is large enough to cover the fish and make a parcel.

Brush each fillet with a little olive oil and top with two slices of lemon, then season with salt and pepper, if required. Fold over the foil to encase the fish. Put the parcels in a roasting tin and bake for 15–20 minutes or until just cooked and opaque.

Meanwhile, to make the salsa, put the tomatoes, shallots, olive oil, garlic, parsley, basil and lemon juice in a bowl. Mix until combined and season to taste with salt and pepper.

Carefully unfold each parcel and arrange the fish and its juices on 4 serving plates. Place a large spoonful of salsa by the side and serve with the asparagus and broccoli.

Prawn and Noodle Stir-fry

Sizzling prawns flash-cooked in sherry with a hint of ginger.

1 tbsp olive oil
2 cloves garlic, finely chopped
2.5 cm (1 inch) ginger, peeled and finely chopped
good splash dry sherry
400 g pack prawns, ready-cooked with shells removed and tails intact
half savoy cabbage, finely shredded

150 g pack thick udon noodles, soaked in boiling water (10 minutes)

In a large heavy-based frying pan, heat the oil and add the garlic and ginger. Cook for about 1 minute, being careful not to burn the garlic. Turn the heat up and pour in the sherry. Bubble for a minute, till the alcohol has cooked away – you will be able to smell this. Throw in the prawns and stir till everything is combined.

Add the cabbage and cook vigorously for about 5 minutes. You want the cabbage to be cooked but still have a crunch. Now stir in the drained noodles and heat through.

Season to taste with sea salt, if required, and freshly ground black pepper. Serve immediately.

DESSERTS

It's a severe regime to live without them, so here are a few recipes to make healthful desserts seem like indulgences (and some indulgences you can say are well . . . tasty).

Cranberry Pear Relish

1 cup brown rice syrup

3 cups fresh cranberries, sorted and rinsed

2 ripe pears, peeled, if desired, and cut into cubes

1/2 teaspoon grated nutmeg

1/2 teaspoon ground allspice

pinch sea salt

2 teaspoons grated lemon zest

Heat the rice syrup in a large saucepan over medium heat until foamy. Add the cranberries, pears, spices and salt. Return to the boil and stir in 1 teaspoon of lemon zest. Reduce the heat and simmer for 25–30 minutes, until the cranberries pop. Transfer to a serving bowl and chill. Before serving, garnish with the remaining lemon zest.

Chocolate Cookies

No one will guess that you have created sinfully delicious treats with healthy ingredients.

1.5 cups rolled oats

1.75 cups wholewheat pastry flour

1/8 teaspoon sea salt

1.5 teaspoons baking powder

1 cup shredded coconut

1/2 cup minced pecans

1 cup brown rice syrup

1/2 cup corn oil

1 cup non-dairy, malt-sweetened chocolate chips (available at natural food stores)

Preheat the oven to 175°C/350°F/Gas Mark 4. Lightly oil a baking sheet. Combine all ingredients, except chocolate, in a large bowl until blended. Gently fold in the chips and drop by spoonfuls onto the prepared baking sheet.

Bake for 18–20 minutes. The cookies should be moist and chewy. Cool on wire racks.

Blueberry and Raspberry Brulée

The vitamin content of the berries remains unaltered by the heat of the grill.

250 g (8 oz) blueberries
250 g (8 oz) raspberries
350 ml (12 fl oz) thick Greek yoghurt or fromage frais
4–6 tablespoons soft brown sugar (oops, don't
 tell anyone)

Mix together the blueberries and raspberries and divide between 4 heatproof dishes or place in 1 large dish.

Spoon the yoghurt or fromage frais over the berries and smooth the top. At this point the puddings can be returned to the fridge to chill overnight or until required.

Sprinkle the sugar over the yoghurt or fromage frais in an even layer and place the dishes on a baking tray. Grill under a preheated grill, close to the heat, for 1–2 minutes or until the sugar has melted and is bubbling in places. Serve immediately.

Viennese Vanilla Crescents

4 cups whole-wheat pastry flour
1/4 teaspoon sea salt
1/4 cup corn oil
1/4 cup brown rice syrup

About 1/2 cup spring or filtered water

1 teaspoon pure vanilla extract

1 teaspoon grated lemon zest

2 cups almonds, ground into a fine meal

2 teaspoons baking powder

About 1/2 cup brown rice syrup, for glaze

Preheat oven to 250°C/400°F/Gas Mark 6. Lightly oil 2 baking sheets.

Combine all ingredients, except 1/4 cup almond meal, in a large bowl. Mix into a stiff dough. Gather into a ball, wrap in waxed paper and refrigerate for 1 hour.

Roll dough into 1/4-inch thick ropes and cut into 2-inch pieces; bend into crescent shapes. Arrange on prepared baking sheets, leaving about 1 inch between cookies.

Bake for 10 minutes. Heat the rice syrup in a saucepan over high heat until it is foamy. While the cookies are still warm, roll in the warm rice syrup and remaining almond meal.

Glazed Apples

4 ripe apples

1 cup apple juice

pinch of sea salt

1 tablespoon kuzu, dissolved in 3 tablespoons cold water

1/2 teaspoon fresh ginger juice (ginger juice is

obtained by finely grating ginger root and
squeezing the juice from the pulp)
Slivered almonds, toasted, for decoration

Preheat oven to 175°C/350°F/Gas Mark 4. Cut the apples in half and remove the cores carefully. Lay the apple halves in a shallow baking dish, cut-side up, and sprinkle with sea salt. Cover and bake for 15 minutes or until tender.

Meanwhile, heat the apple juice over low heat until hot. Stir in the dissolved kuzu and cook, stirring, until the mixture thickens and clears, 3–4 minutes. Add the ginger juice and pour over the cooked apples. Increase oven heat to 200°C/400°F/Gas Mark 6. Return the apples to the oven, uncovered, for 15 minutes to set glaze. Serve warm, sprinkled with almonds, if desired.

JUICING

One of the best ways to make use of the nutrients in fruit and vegetables is to make your own fresh juices. It is, after all, a lot easier to drink a glass of carrot juice than munch your way through a bag of carrots. In addition, the body absorbs nutrients from liquid foods more rapidly and efficiently than if they are taken in the form of mineral and vitamin supplements.

The World Health Organization has said that vitamins A (beta-carotene from vegetable sources), C and E are vital for health. These vitamins, together with the minerals, selenium and zinc, are known antioxidants. One of the many benefits of juicing, alongside cleansing and healing and renewed energy, is that you get all the vitamin content of the fruit.

The trick to effective use of juices is to make them fresh and to have them between meals or in place of a meal. Juices can be made from almost any fruit or vegetable imaginable, giving you a power-packed nutritional drink with a wide range of health-protecting properties.

Smoothies

Smoothies are thick juice drinks. You can use them as a meal replacement if you want or as a pick-me-up in the morning or afternoon. You can be as adventurous as you wish with your smoothies. Fruit is the most important ingredient of the smoothie. To thicken the drink you can use bananas, unflavoured yoghurt, or you can add soymilk for a smooth texture. Isn't it wonderful to see so many juice bars opening up in cities and airports that now allow us the choice to opt for a delicious nutritious drink or a Diet Coke!

Berry Amazing

Strawberries, raspberries, blackberries, blueberries, blackcurrants and redcurrants are among my favourites and are all packed with antioxidants. They are very cleansing and, ultimately, have an anti-ageing effect. Strawberries are also thought to be beneficial for the skin – smoothing out lines and wrinkles – and for soothing arthritic inflammation. Raspberries are a mild laxative and good, too, for indigestion.

Many berries also contain high levels of minerals, especially calcium, magnesium and potassium. Food processors and blenders don't do the job as well as a juicing machine, so invest in one – your body will love you for it. All the best intentions can easily go out of the window unless things are to hand. So stockpile fruits, vegetables and other foods that you will be using every day. Set yourself up to be healthy, plan well.

Detox Juice

This is a good morning energizer containing beetroot, one of the most effective liver-cleansing vegetables.

2 dessert apples

115 g (4 oz) white seedless grapes

1 large carrot

55 g (2 oz) cooked beetroot in natural juices

1 cm (1/2 inch) piece of fresh root ginger

Quarter the apples and then put them through a juicer along with the grapes, carrot, beetroot and ginger. Serve immediately.

Spring Into Action

1 orange, peeled
handful of strawberries
3 carrots, topped and tailed
1 lemon, peeled
sprinkle of wheatgerm
handful of ice, if you wish

Once all the ingredients are juice, stir in the wheatgerm and pour into a glass over ice.

Very Green Juice

2 sticks celery
half small cucumber
3 royal gala apples
2.5 cm (1 inch) fresh ginger
2 cups spinach
half small pineapple, peeled
half lemon, peeled
flesh of 1 ripe avocado

Juice everything apart from the avocado and ice. Pour the juice into a blender along with the ice and avocado and give a good whiz.

Creating A Healthy Home

Dear Marlene,

As you know, I have for some time been a believer in a healthy lifestyle, but found it difficult to put into practice. However, you have inspired me to eat healthily, and my once cynical husband, George has now converted to a 'well-being' lifestyle and delights in telling friends about our "wellness home". George has always exercised, but had a poor diet, and would push his vegetables aside in favour of bread, creamy sauces and cheese. Now knowing the importance of a well balanced diet, he eats the veg that I make, and takes his nutritional supplements religiously every day. I feel more energised and have an even greater zest for life he tells me.

It is so easy to get the children to eat healthily now, with your encouragement. Jonathan doesn't like soups with 'bits' so I puree them and that disguises that he is eating spinach and watercress, or peppers and tomatoes, he just thinks it's mummy's yummie soup. Very clever Marlene!

The kids now love to make their own smoothies packed with berries, as they know the value of the antioxidants. You have certainly made a difference to what we eat and

Jonathan now eats more veggies and fruit, and less sweeties AND he even eats porridge with berries and honey. Chloe who was a much healthier eater is delighted her brother now has the same diet as her.

As well as influencing our eating habits, you also enhanced our sleep when you introduced us to our Kenkodream Magnetic Sleep System. Well done in convincing George, the cynic, that this sleep system would improve our sleeping pattern. He actually changes the pillow to a conventional one at weekends, as he says that 'Marlene's' Pillow wakes me up too early, too full of energy and zest. I also love my magnetic sleep mask and I am sure that along with good nutrition is what helped me to make a very quick recovery from eye surgery to remove cataracts.

Nutritionists are always telling us that water is essential for well being. It is reassuring to know that we are drinking 'quality' water from our Pi Mag System. I use it for everything, making soups, cooking vegetables, and my plants love it also. They are thriving.

Thank you for everything Marlene, you have certainly put your mark on the Thompson household.

Best Wishes

Janice Thompson

Recipes Toolbox

Have fun in the kitchen. Try and make the energy in your kitchen one of lightness, joy and creativity. If your kitchen looks dark and forbidding, cheer it up. Paint it a light colour, get new curtains, clean it out and throw out the junk.

Your recipe is a map, not the territory. Use the ideas from any recipe book and convert them. As you get used to using some of the foods we have been talking about, you will find that you can convert most of your favourite recipes using some new ingredients.

Get good equipment. Try to get the best kitchen implements you can, especially the pots. Good food needs attention and if you are cooking more of your food from scratch, you need pots with thicker bottoms. Try to stay away from the non-stick varieties or aluminium – there is concern that they out-gas chemicals into the food. For sure, food cooked in aluminium takes on the taste of the pan. I know, you don't want to be a fanatic. Do what works for you.

Gas is best.

If you have a heart condition, use less salt.

If you have kids, experiment and find out the healthy things they like.

Cook with love, eat with gratitude.

CHAPTER SEVEN
MOVE IT OR LOSE IT

Exercise is an important part of what I do. Regardless of what kind of a problem a person has, if they can move any part of their body, exercise will make them feel better. Here's an interesting fact. More and more people every year complain of tiredness and yet we have less physical activity than any generation before us. What's happening? Very few people I know have jobs that are physically taxing. I know those jobs exist and would sympathize with someone who was tired after lifting, digging or building all day. The truth is that a lack of exercise makes us more, not less, tired.

Our understanding of the importance of exercise and what really works has changed drastically over the past fifteen years. When I was doing high-impact aerobics in the 80s, it was considered to be the best thing going. Well, the idea of improving cardiovascular and aerobic health was good, but the techniques were misguided. Pounding a body to the point of exhaustion is not only unproductive, it can be hurtful. I damaged both my knees and know many people who have had the same experience doing high impact exercises or working with weights.

There is no reason that extreme punishment has to be experienced for good health. This is true in both exercise and diet. The same way that some people think that healthy food has to taste bad, some feel that they can't be getting any benefit from exercise if there is no pain. What is known now is that the exercises that do the most lasting good are those that create moderate improvement over time. Usually they are the activities that are simple and can be done by anyone. Even if you need some instruction to begin with, they can be done without complicated equipment (or even without any equipment).

As the median age of the population rises, the number of middle-aged people doing exercise has increased radically. The reason for this is simple, it can add years onto your life – literally. A European Union study found that 40% of 40–50-year-olds exercise at least twice a week. In America 57 million people now exercise 100 days a year. They do it to recover from illness, to avoid getting sick and just for the enjoyment.

If we do not exercise regularly a number of predictable events take place. Part of the ageing process is the stiffening of tendons and ligaments. This inhibits the range of motion and makes us more prone to injury. A regular exercise programme flexes these connective tissues. Bones start to become more brittle after forty years of age unless strengthened by exercise. Cardiovascular capacity and response declines with age unless we are engaged in regular activity. The picture is pretty sad. If you don't use it, you lose it.

Most of the people who come to me for training have difficulty with exercise the first week or so; some even feel physically sick. They complain they don't have the energy. After a couple of weeks they notice that instead of feeling tired after training, they feel invigorated. This is a very common result – any trainer will tell you the same. The reasons are simple.

The body is designed to move. When we don't move, the body loses muscle, endurance, co-ordination, flexibility, the capacity to relax and aerobic condition. Each of these things is essential for good health and the enjoyment of life. When we look at the specifics, it's amazing that so many can stay alive with such little activity. The fact is that aside from diet there is nothing more important than exercise for physical health.

Just consider for a moment the benefits of healthy lungs. When we are performing useful exercise (more on this later), we increase the amount of oxygen in the body. Oxygen is one of our most important nutrients. When we increase oxygen, the body and mind improve dramatically in function. Other nutrients are used more efficiently and we increase our capacity to relax.

The heart deserves a special mention here too. The heart is a muscle. Like all muscles it becomes stronger when exercised. When the heart is not challenged it becomes flaccid and unable to cope with dramatic changes in blood chemistry, emotion or physical demand. Studies have shown that in combination with a healthy diet, exercise can bring health back to men and women who have suffered severe cardiac challenges.

Aside from lungs and heart, another system worth mentioning here is the lymphatic system. Lymph vessels and lymph nodes are connected to the spleen. This system creates white blood cells and has a very important function in protecting the body from infection and disease. Interestingly there is no pump on the lymphatic system as in the circulatory system. The best way to invigorate and move lymph through the body is when we exercise. People who exercise regularly seem to have a greater resistance to disease.

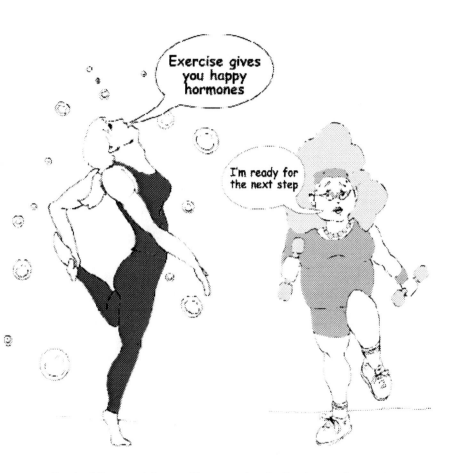

Part of the problem with exercise is that people tend to think of it as work. The only work is getting started and keeping it up for the first month; after that you will be doing it because it makes you feel good. Not exercising at all is simply a very bad habit. It is a self-fulfilling prophecy: "I'm too tired, I can't get up off the couch, it's hopeless." Guess what? When the lazy old flaccid monkey that operates this mantra shows up, its always true. The more you sit on the couch, the less likely you'll be to get up. It takes one superhuman lunge to change it all.

This is not about having "fabulous abs in ten days" or "losing twenty pounds in a week". It's all about being healthy, enjoying life, being able to play with the kids or grandkids, and feeling enlivened instead of over the hill. It's not about looking like a model or a movie star, we have way too much of that. In fact, that's part of the problem.

Advertising and the media bury us with an avalanche of images showing us what is handsome, beautiful and desirable. It has lead us to a situation where women and an increasing number of men either try to starve and stuff themselves into a mould they never will fit, or simply give up and sink into the couch. This is not healthy. You can weigh more than you should and still be fit, you can lack perfectly sculpted muscles and still have vitality and flexibility. Fitness is not just for the wealthy or the person blessed with a good physique at birth. Let's look at some simple things we can all do. You don't have to buy a Lycra outfit either.

I am going to introduce you to the things I have used to best effect. There are many more and you should experiment as you get into step. Find those things that work for you. It doesn't need to be complicated. Doing something like walking or riding a bike every day is more effective than going to a fancy gym once a week. Do things that you can fit into your life; doing something is better than doing nothing. Don't sabotage your self. Did you know that most health clubs would go broke if people only paid when they went? Most people buy the membership card then stay home. Garages all over the world are filled with exercise equipment bought in a rush of enthusiasm and left to rust.

Going for a Walk

Most experts agree that as little as thirty minutes of moderate exercise, five days a week, will keep a person with a healthy diet at a good fitness level. Ten thousand steps per day will keep you fit and healthy. Most people can do that. It requires no equipment, can be done in the country or the city and I swear by it. It is low impact and can be done by both the young and the old. Once you start you will get hooked because you feel energized.

You may have to re-write the rulebook to get stepping out. Spend less time in front of the television, or surfing the Internet for starters. When folks tell me they can't fit fitness into their lives, I always ask them this question: "How many hours do you spend watching television?"

Muscle loss occurs very slowly, easily giving the impression that lack of activity isn't affecting you. In reality, this loss of muscle strength ends up affecting all aspects of your life. Muscles are what gives your body the ability to move and supports your skeleton, giving you freedom and independence to do the things you want to do in life. Disuse results in poor posture, limited range of motion around the joints, and loss of strength. Strength-training exercises are necessary to prevent this muscle wasting. Placing stress on the muscles forces them to become stronger over time instead of weaker. It is never too late to start.

Make walking a part of your daily routine. Remember that the best time for you to go for a walk is always the time that is most convenient for you. It doesn't have to be a discipline – use the stairs instead of the lift and walk instead of using the car when making short trips.

Find yourself a walking buddy. Go with a friend and set some goals for yourselves, increasing your mileage each week. It's a good time to catch up with each other rather than chatting on the phone. Why not schedule long walks at the weekend so that you can get out in nature. Go to the beach or mountains and make your exercise fun to do, something you look forward to rather than resist.

Muscle needs calories to survive. The more you build muscle, the faster you will lose weight and the better it will stay off. The more muscle you have, the speedier the metabolism. Simply put, bigger muscles burn more calories than smaller ones, even during sleep. Remember, a total fitness programme includes warming up, stretching, strength training and some sort of cardiovascular activity for heart health and extra body fat burning. Whatever your objectives, start out slowly.

The older you get, the harder it is to maintain your weight by simply restricting what you eat. Exercise is essential to weight loss as you age. Walking briskly for half an hour daily not only consumes a couple of hundred calories, it boosts your metabolic rate for the rest of the day. Just walking has been proven to improve the following health problems:

Heart Disease – Brisk walking is known to be good for the heart, which makes a lot of sense. The heart is a muscle, after all, and anything that makes the blood flow faster through a muscle helps keep it in shape.

Stroke – In a recent study it was found that 20 or more hours per week decreased the risk of stroke by 40%.

Diabetes – Studies provide evidence that brisk walking for 30 minutes a day can postpone and even prevent the development of type 2 diabetes in people who are overweight and whose bodies have already started having trouble metabolizing glucose.

Osteoporosis – Walking not only strengthens the muscles but also builds up the bones to which they are attached.

Arthritis – Walking reduces the pain by strengthening the muscles around the joint.

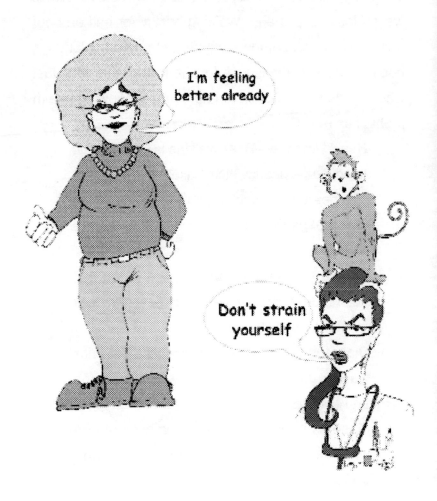

SUPER WALKING

Several years ago I discovered weighted trainers. The best on the market are called Cardiostrides; I have given information about them in the products section at the end of the book. You need training shoes that are designed well or they will give undue pressure on the knees and can cause problems. If the design is right they will make you stand up straight and reduce knee strain.

The effect of weighted trainers is that they maximize the cardiovascular effect of your walk and increase metabolism. A 20-minute walk gives you similar benefits to a 30-minute walk. I love them and my clients rave about the difference they make.

They look like normal trainers but have different weight options. By using different insoles (inserts) you can adjust the weight.

You give yourself a much more intense workout by using them for your walking programme. They strengthen and tone the legs, hips, butts and abs and strengthen the postural muscles in the lower back. Keep your posture looking good. Cardiostrides give you a fat-burning, cardiovascular and muscle-toning workout just by walking. They intensify the benefits of what you do. It is best to start off with short time spans when you start until your legs get used to the workout.

Meridian Stretches

Earlier I talked a little bit about "chi", the concept of life energy found in Chinese medicine and philosophy. As the ancient practice of this medicine and health care developed, the Chinese discovered that life energy moves in a particular pattern. They observed that the energy flowed like ribbons of light through the body and nourished the organs and tissues as it moved. I think of these ribbons as electrical wires. The energy for this system comes to us through the chi in the food we eat, the air we breathe, the water we drink, our environment and even other people. If the energy is too high or too low the lines get blocked or start to decay. That's why the right choices are important. Good energy keeps the lines open, no static.

These electric lines are called "meridians" in acupuncture. They circulate energy through the body and need stimulation. All of traditional Chinese medicine is aimed to balance this flow. It can be done by stimulating or sedating the meridian with needles as in acupuncture, by applying specific pressure to the skin through Shiatsu massage or through movement and exercise.

The stretches below are some that I use in my work to get the whole system of chi in the body moving and rebalanced. Give them a try and see what happens.

Remember, it may take several weeks or months to

achieve these positions. Always warm up the body prior to stretching. Pay attention to what your body tells you, it will guide you. Better still; join a local yoga class for personal instruction.

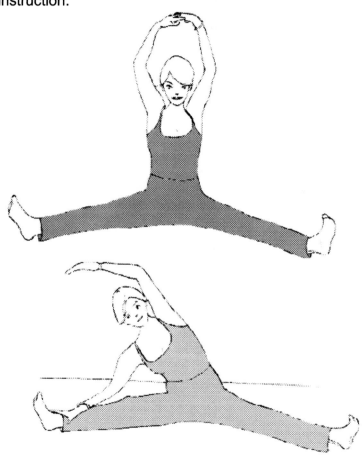

Liver/Gallbladder Meridian Stretch

Sit on the floor with your legs as wide apart as is comfortable. With your back straight and hands together, stretch your arms over your head and take a deep breath.

Slowly exhale as you stretch forward gently towards your right foot or calf, aiming to reach the toes.

Never over-stretch, instead relax into a comfortable stretch, at the same time taking deep breaths, let the body relax into the stretch and as you hold the stretch the muscles will start to lengthen. You will feel the stretch along the outside of your right leg and the inside of your left. Repeat twice, then slowly bring your body back into an upright position and repeat on the left side.

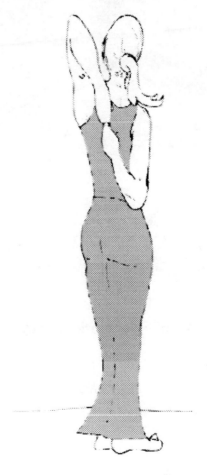

Heart/Small Intestine Meridian Stretch

Sit on the floor with your knees open and the soles of the feet together. Keep your back straight. Take your right hand over your shoulder and take the left arm behind the back of your waist, reaching upwards until you are touching your fingers with the right hand. Aim to point your elbow towards the ceiling. Change and repeat on the left side.

Stomach/Spleen Meridian Stretch

Start gradually and, as your muscles become stronger, you can increase the intensity of this stretch. Kneel on the floor and place your hands either side. Keeping your spine straight, inhale and put the weight on your hands. Exhale and push your hips towards the ceiling at the same time as dropping your head back and resting the elbows on the floor; try and relax into the position. You will feel the stretch running down the front of your thighs and torso. Take five deep breaths in this position. Gently, using your hands, push your body back into the starting position.

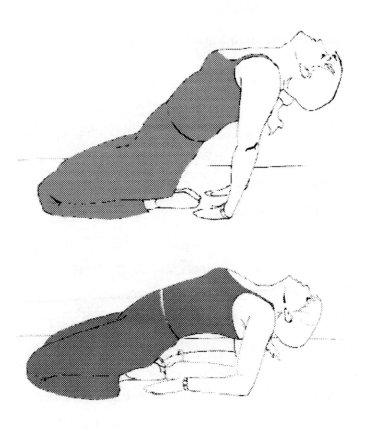

Lungs/Large Intestine Meridian Stretch

Standing upright, clasp your hands behind your back and gently begin to bend forward, keeping your knees unlocked. Raise your arms as high as possible behind you. Hold the position and breathe deeply for 5 breaths. Come back to the start position and repeat three times. Many of us become stiff and inflexible in the upper body and you may find your arms won't stretch very far, but with practice this is a super stretch to perform.

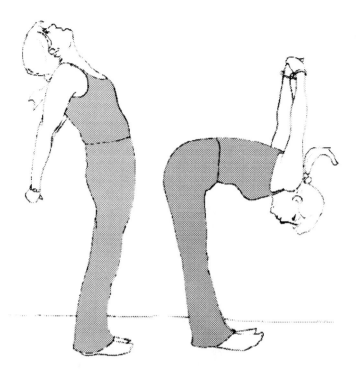

Kidney/Bladder Meridian Stretch

We must move the muscles at the back of the thighs and this is a fantastic stretch to help lengthen those tight hamstrings. Sit on the floor and stretch your legs out in front of you; keeping the knees relaxed and your lower back straight, gently stretch forwards, taking your hands towards your toes or to the knees or ankles and relax into the position with deep breaths; gently, with each breath, visualize the muscles softening and relaxing, allowing you to stretch further with each breath. You may also perform this stretch standing if you prefer. Hang forward with the knees soft and let the arms hang loosely, aiming to reach for the toes.

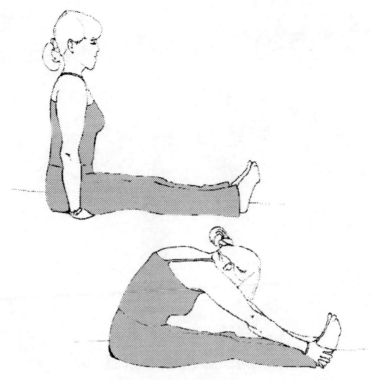

Exercise Your Mind

Exercise doesn't just benefit the body. Did you ever notice that if you have an argument or are out of sorts, you can just walk if off? Movement shifts your energy in a good way. Exercise regularly and you'll feel more optimistic, with a more hopeful outlook on life in general. Now isn't that worth getting in a sweat over. I teach the Chi Ball Method: we use a holistic approach to exercise that incorporates Tai Chi, Yoga, Pilates and Deep Relaxation. We modify the programme to fit with the seasons. I like this approach and love the variety of approaches we use.

If you want to move past walking and stretching, I recommend that you find a good teacher. In most advanced approaches such as tai chi, yoga or Pilates, it is important that you know how to do the exercises properly so that you don't injure yourself.

The Spirit of Tai Chi

Historians place the beginning of tai chi somewhere in the eleventh century, but its origins probably lie further back in history. Much like yoga, tai chi developed into a holistic approach to living in balance with nature. From its early association with the martial arts it has grown a following that recognize the health benefits of doing this daily "energy dance". Tai chi is built around the body in motion.

The forms of tai chi emphasize soft, flowing, circular movements. Each position moves seamlessly into the next. Tai chi is excellent for gaining flexibility and balance. It improves circulation and co-ordination, and helps relax and strengthen the muscular and nervous system. The feet are always firmly on the ground, movements intrinsically beautiful and at the same time charged with symbolic meaning. Movements of the muscles represent movements of the consciousness.

Tai chi connects the mind and the body through the breath and is a wonderful way to 'feel' the chi (energy) moving through your body.

Like yoga, I have seen many athletes who scoff at the lack of "punch" in doing these exercises that are Eastern in origin. They say that there is not enough muscle burn in doing something so slowly. They say that until they try them out and then feel embarrassed to find out that they can't do the exercises. The reason that these practices have been around for hundreds of years is because they work!

Yoga

The practice of yoga may go back over 3,000 years in the area that is now Pakistan and India. As in many cultures, people knew that if they were to remain healthy it was important to have flexibility. The word "yoga" means "union" or "joining". Traditional yoga was more a way of life than a series of exercises. It encompassed exercise, meditation, social behaviour, diet and the whole range of human activity.

Two major concepts in yoga teach the importance of breath to vitality and clear thinking, and that flexibility is the best cure for ageing. For many years yoga was seen only as a new-age fad; it is now recognized as physically therapeutic. Studies have shown that a wide range of common complaints, such as backache, hypertension and migraine headaches, can be greatly helped by yoga exercises.

Old age begins when we allow the joints and spine to stiffen. When we say that someone looks "younger than their age", it usually has to do with the way they move. Through a variety of yoga poses (called asanas), you will feel how to let the pressures go and rediscover the flexibility that is still there. You will find that this flexibility will flow out into all areas of your life; your gain in yoga is much more than just physical. Flexibility keeps your joints open and organs young. Flexibility is life. Stiffness is death. The slang word for a corpse is in fact a "stiff".

Yoga teaches us that "prana" is the essential life force that glues the cells together. Without the presence of prana the body decomposes and dies. Yoga really works and the ultimate aim is unity and balance. What fun I have had teaching this to many clients. Trying a tree pose for the first time, for instance, for many is hysterical; they fall about laughing and some look as if they have been on the cooking sherry. A few weeks of patience and better vision of what they are aiming for and, wow! It's amazing every time to see the sense of accomplishment and pleasure when someone reaches a new peak of physical fitness. Remember when you were learning to ride a bicycle, it got easier as you went along? If you haven't had the wonderful experience of yoga, you should try it, because while you have breath you have hope, so put your hope into action. Your body will love you for it. There are yoga classes offered all over the UK. Find a chi ball instructor or a yoga teacher who you like and try a few trial classes.

Pilates

Many of the injuries and disabilities of today are caused by our modern machine-oriented society. Repetitive movements on computers and sitting for hours at a desk contradict the physiological needs of the human body. Pilates was originally designed for use by dancers. The exercises prepared them for the kind of extreme demands that professional dancers require. If you desire a flat stomach, a longer, leaner body and wonderful posture, try Pilates. The main emphasis is on elongating the body to create a longer, leaner silhouette. As with the rest of the chi ball philosophies, Pilates movements integrate the mind and body.

The slow, controlled movements enable energy to move more freely throughout the body. There is no need for overexertion, it's about quality not quantity. Pilates is great for mobility and endurance; it targets weak, under-utilized muscles in the abdomen, lower back, arms and legs.

This uncomplicated series of exercises is focused on strengthening the core muscles. These are the muscles that are so important in maintaining back health and general fitness. They emphasize strengthening the smaller muscles, which can give you the shape that you want. You can tone your stomach, thighs and arms, reshape your buttocks and get your self into that thong (male and female). One question for you all! How do you feel when you stand naked in front of the mirror? Like what you see? If not, you are never too old to start a new exercise programme. Find a chi ball instructor or join a Pilates class.

Office Yoga.
Exercises to do in the office or at home.

Tone your buttocks! You can do this one anywhere, sitting, standing at the bus stop, waiting in a queue at the supermarket. Clench the muscles in your buttocks, hold for a count of five, then slowly relax. Do as many times as you wish.

Bat wing arms (or cheerio's) as we call them. When you wave to someone you don't want the bottom of your arm wobbling around. These arm circles are great for getting rid of this unwanted area of loose skin. Sit up straight with your arms out to the side, palms upwards. Slowly make circles with your hands.

Tone your bust. Sit up straight and put your hands together as if you were praying. Push the palms together as hard as you can. Count to ten and repeat as many times as you can.

Get the circulation moving. Circle your feet and ankles 20 times on each foot. Rotate both clockwise and then anti clockwise. Remember the feet are the framework of the whole body and it feels great to feel the heat moving there. Next, stretch out your leg and point and flex your foot to work out your calf muscles

Lengthen your neck. This is great for relieving the stress in your shoulders. Drop your head forward taking your chin to your chest. Very slowly bring it back up imagining your cervical spine in a string of pearls and you are stacking the pearls one at a time.

Strengthen the arms. Use the arms of your chair (not a rolling one) to support you as you place your hands, fingers facing forward, and raise your bottom as if to stand up then bend the elbows to take you back down to the starting position. (keep your elbows tucked in to your waist with each repetition) Repeat ten times slowly and synchronise your breath with the movement, as you breathe in go up, as you exhale go down.

Tension releases. Stretch upwards spreading your fingers as wide as possible. Look up at the ceiling and stretch for a count of five clenching your fists, release the fingers and bring the arms back to starting position. Repeat ten times.

Clasp your hands above your head, and stretch towards the ceiling. From your waist, bend to the right, keeping your arms stretched and breathe. Return to the centre and stretch to the left.

Place your hands on the arms of your chair and breathe in, from the waist look behind you to the right, as far as you can, breathing out - then repeat to the left.

If you really want to cheer up your colleagues try a facial exercise or two. That will raise a few smiles in the office. Grin as widely as you can (really over exaggerate the grin) and hold for a count of five. Repeat ten times.

The other facial exercise that my clients have a good laugh at themselves is by opening your mouth into a big O shape, now pull the top lip over the teeth (without using your hands) and wrinkle your nose up and down like a rabbit, great for plumping up the cheeks and the nasal labial lines.

Deep Relaxation and Visualization

Letting go of the tension in every muscle is an integral part of all the above philosophies. Due to poor postural habits, excessive strain is placed on various muscle groups, which causes pain. Relaxation and pain relief may be elusive, even during sleep. All too often we turn to the quick-fix method of drugs and alcohol for relief. It is important to know how to relax fully.

Preparing for relaxation is important. Find a nice comfy space and take the phone off the hook. Lie down on the floor with the body's weight comfortably supported. Place a small cushion under the head to lengthen the back of the neck and, if you wish, tuck yourself in with a light blanket. Let the feet and knees drop open to the sides, have your palms turned upwards, let the abdominal muscles sink down toward the spine. Relax the face muscles and the jaw, let the tongue relax in the floor of the mouth (if you are anything like me – I like a wee chat – it will have been well used all day). Start to name the parts of the body to yourself as you work up from the feet through the legs, torso, arms, neck and head. (You know the leg bone's connected to the thigh bone.) As you move up the body, relax each part as you go. When I finish typing this chapter, I'm off to do just that.

Slowing down allows for higher levels of awareness so that you'll know what's right for your unique self. Relaxation allows you to experience full-body consciousness. Allow your mind to travel through the body to release excess tension so that there can be a free flow of "chi" through the body and the mind. Let your mind touch your body. Let your body respond in healing and well being.

When I end a session, I always relax in this manner. In the winter months my clients bring a blanket and I light some candles; they place their chi ball at the back of their necks and slowly, with the eyes closed, take their heads from side to side to bring themselves into balance. It is perfect to do this right after stretching and limbering the joints. This is my favourite part. I find this interesting as so many of us don't like stillness, or to be in this space, of relaxation. If you try this for the first time and can't switch your mind off (i.e. you're too busy thinking about what you need at Asda on the way home), have patience, it doesn't happen overnight. It truly is wonderful to "feel" the whole body completely soften and for your mind to dictate this.

I get my clients to focus on different parts of the body where there is stress and imagine that they are breathing into and out of that area. Being aware and being conscious of your breath is the best way to start any relaxation session. Notice how breath is movement, movement is life, life is movement, breath is life. Sometimes clients fall asleep because they are so relaxed. There are so many ways and methods to do deep relaxation and perhaps you may wish to purchase a CD or tape on relaxation to get you started. Even better, make a tape for yourself, slowly talking you through the body. Enjoy the full experience.

Skin Brushing

When you are exercising regularly you may notice that your skin becomes softer. The skin is the largest organ in the body that has excretory functions. Pores get blocked, fatty tissue keeps old skin in place and the skin can't breathe. Self-massage and skin brushing helps the body to discharge toxins that build up in the skin. The gentle brushing stimulates the lymphatic system and opens up the pores. It is one of the best lymphatic cleansers known, and therefore is supportive to the spleen. When practised daily for a few months it can also improve body tone. This treatment should be carried out on dry skin for about 3 minutes prior to having a shower or bath.

1. Brush the soles as well as the upper sides of the feet using a long-handled natural bristle brush with soft or medium bristles. With long, sweeping strokes, brush up the legs, covering all of the skin's surface area, concentrating on the thighs and buttocks. There is no need to brush hard, it should be a pleasant feeling.

2. Put one arm up in the air, allowing gravity to help drain the lymph to the armpit and sweep down the arm with gentle strokes, drawing the brush towards the armpit.

3. Brush the torso by brushing towards the heart; when doing the lower abdomen, brush up the right-hand side, just on the inside of the hip bone, across the transverse colon beneath the ribs and down the left-hand side, then gently across the pelvic area to complete the

circle. This follows the natural direction of the colon. Repeat.

4. When working near the breast area, brush over the top of the breast, always aiming for the armpit – and remember, be gentle with over-sensitive areas!

5. Your skin will become more resilient and you will be able to take more vigorous brushing after a few weeks. Visualize while you do this that your body is being cleansed and purified. It is best to follow a regular daily programme of skin brushing once to twice a day for three months, then reduce this to twice a week – preferably keeping to a regular routine.

6. The *piece de resistance* is to take a warm shower and follow this with a quick blast of cold water. Apart from being highly stimulating, this encourages the dilation and contraction of the blood vessels and further incites movement of the lymph. You will feel very invigorated.

Try this. Clench your fists really tight. Now clench your jaw. Hold the tension as long as you can and then release it. Now imagine that you were walking around every day with your muscles bunched up like that. That's the way many of us live. Stress in the body becomes chronic. Energy gets blocked and we get used to it.

Almost everyone has a pattern of held energy; some people call it "armouring". The body becomes twisted around these stress patterns and we feel worn out just by holding them. In energy medicine these patterns are significant. When we are healthy we move with a certain grace, no matter how old we are. When the body is relaxed and energy is balanced, we are less prone to accidents and injury. We have greater energy because we aren't wasting it.

When you exercise regularly you start to become more aware of the life force in your body. You realize that when you are walking freely, doing yoga or tai chi, that it is almost as if your body disappears, you are just floating. (Don't call for the men in the white coats – it's true.) Ask trained athletes about this and they will tell you that most of them experience this. Some call it being "in the zone" or "in the flow". They are experiencing the life force in action.

The study of tai chi, yoga, dance and most martial arts aim at enhancing this life force and learning to move it in the body. Many good athletes use visualization in this way. They imagine themselves performing at a peak level, they train their body and then when they are competing, they can just relax and enjoy the activity.

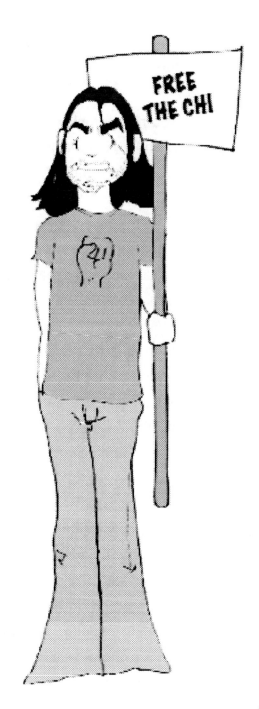

Elaine Learns to Breathe

Dear Marlene,

In a nutshell, you have simply changed my life. You are my conscience and my life coach. I regularly suffered from IBS, migraine, and acid reflux. I found it difficult to relax. You talked to me about the effect this would have on my long-term health, especially as we are all living longer. Initially, I became a regular at your Chi Ball Classes and found the methods used had a really positive effect on my mental and physical well-being.

First of all I had to learn how to breathe, which was a bit of a shock as I thought I had been doing ok all of these years, then I had to learn to concentrate on the movements and the meditation. For the first time in years, I felt really chilled out after class. Soon after I was sleeping better and not feeling tired when I woke up.

You then focused on my eating habits and had quite a time convincing me of the benefits of miso soup and the myriad of beans and pulses on offer. However, it really is miraculous the difference food can make. You have taught me that the best thing I can do for my body is to nourish it properly and take care of it rather than neglect it for years as most of us do and are then somewhat surprised when we suffer ill health. Your philosophy is so simple and makes sense and has worked for me. I am done with the medication and ailments that I suffered for a very long time.

Elaine Dunlop
Bank of Scotland

Inspiration Runs Deep

Dear Marlene,

As someone who does not enjoy, or particularly like to exercise I must say that I have been inspired so much by your Chi Ball Classes and actually have fun as well as working every organ and muscle in my body when I come. I feel my energy levels have increased since I started and that is why I continue to be a regular participant.

When I miss my classes due to other engagements, my energy is always lower so I know how much they work and how much I benefit from them.

I have also noticed how much healthier I feel and again see the difference in my energy since sleeping on my magnetic sleep system and taking your advice and drinking more water throughout the day. If it works for me, it will work for anyone.

Thank you Marlene for teaching me about 'Energy Medicine' I love it.

With thanks
Susan Stern

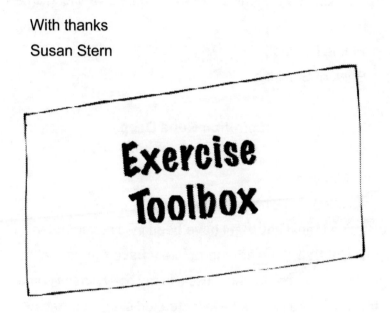

So let's review a few simple things about exercise that can help get us on our way.

Do the simple things first. You don't need to be complicated or attend a class to start exercising. Just get up and get out. Start with a simple time limit or distance and then increase it a little every four days or so. Set yourself goals to double up your first attempt. You want to feel a sense of accomplishment – you deserve it, you are doing something good for yourself.

Get a buddy. It is always more fun to exercise with someone else and it provides extra motivation. Make a commitment to each other to stay with a set schedule with concrete goals. You can decide to walk together three or four times a week and set a goal to double your distance every two weeks. After two months you can decide if the experiment was worth it.

Warm up and stretch thoroughly. Learn some simple stretching exercises and do them before you workout. This will eliminate injury and ensure that you maximize the effect of what you do.

Increase strengthening exercises slowly. If you decide to use weights, go slowly and concentrate on repetitions rather than increasing the weight too soon. You will still build muscle but it will be flexible muscle and you will reduce the prospect of injury.

CHAPTER EIGHT
REST AND RELAXATION

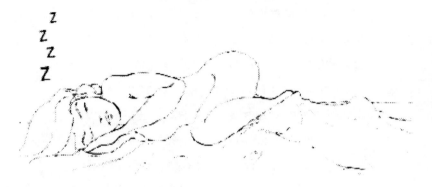

In today's world it often feels like we are racing the clock to get everything done. This is one of the major causes of stress. It almost seems as if there were fewer hours in the day than there were in the past. One of the things I often hear from my clients is that they don't have enough time to be healthy. That's an interesting thought. What it really means is that they are spending their time getting sick. Just a little review of some of the things we have already covered is good here.

Remember when I said that stress is what happens when we ask our body and mind to do things that we are not designed to do? Well that wasn't really the whole story. Sometimes we can do all that is demanded of us, but only if we do one thing at a time. I can talk on the phone, I can drive the car, I can pay attention to the baby in the back seat – I just can't do them all at once and do them well.

Dealing with a stressful life is sometimes just a question of doing one thing at a time.

If I am talking with someone or doing something important I don't need to answer the phone. That is why I have an answering machine. When we try to do too much at the same time the mind tries its best to keep up. Often the message that's communicated to the body is anxiety. Anxiety is the close cousin of fear and this is important to remember.

In Chinese medicine, fear is associated with the functioning of the kidneys and the adrenal glands. The adrenals are the key to a lot of what we see as stress. It is the fight or flight response running wild. When the mind is close to panic the body thinks there is something to fear. When there is too much information to process it can create anxiety and even panic. The irony is that many of the things we do when stressed out create more stress or further weaken the adrenals. Here are two self-medications that don't work.

Eating for your stress is a common strategy that makes the problem worse. When we are stressed there is a tendency to eat comfort foods, things that distract us with taste or texture. These foods are invariably sugar rich. Everything from sticky sweets to alcohol is a possibility. These are foods that produce a sugar rush and then leave us heavy and more dissatisfied than before. Welcome to the merry-go-round. When we are not well nourished the body becomes more acidic. This acidic condition affects our nervous system and brain function, which sets us up for more stress.

Drinking coffee is a popular stress option. Coffee sits right next to cigarettes as a really bad idea when you are stressed out. What is happening is that we are using something that gives us a temporary illusion of focus and undermines our long-term ability to function. In fact, a coffee and a cigarette is almost the signature image of someone who thrives on stress. We might as well have a little battery acid and inhale car exhaust for all the good it does us. Each of us has a stress cycle. We feel the pressure, we try to keep up and then we try to break out by doing something. This is natural but only helps if we are doing something that creates a better cycle than the one we have.

Breaking Stress Cycles

Most people who exercise regularly will tell you that it is one of the best ways to reduce or banish stress in your life. It is a counter-intuitive action because stress usually makes us tired. When we are finished with the stressful activity we want to curl up in the corner and be left alone. When you are stressed, try breaking it by taking a short walk.

Take a ten-minute walk in the coffee break or go for a walk at lunch and have a smaller meal. If you are following the advice in chapter seven, you will be feeling less stress already.

Desktop Meditation

Sit quietly, feet on the floor, sitting comfortably in an upright position. Close your eyes and slowly withdraw your mind from outside stimulation while maintaining awareness and wakefulness. Silently do a body inventory. Visualize every part of your body, starting with your feet, moving up through your legs, belly, chest, arms, neck and head. As you do this, slowly tense each area so that at the end your whole body is tensed. Now reverse the process, relaxing every part as if it were sand running out of a sack or water leaking out of a pond. This only takes a few minutes to do right in your living room or at your desk. Now breathe very slowly and softly through the nose and exhale through the mouth. Concentrate your mind on your breath. If your concentration wanders, bring it back to your breath.

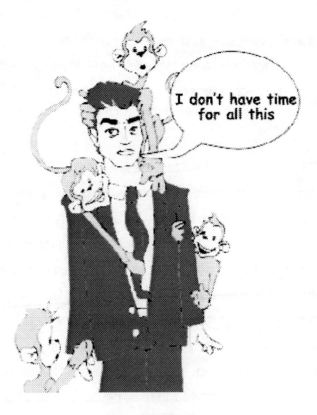

The Big Self

Start as before, sitting in a relaxed position. For this exercise a quiet room is best but not necessary. Start with a total body inventory as before, but without the tension. Just be aware of the space your body occupies. When you are aware of your whole body, stretch your awareness out to encompass the immediate space around you in the room. Keep coming back to yourself and then flexing your imagination out to encompass the whole room. As you become more proficient at this, you can imagine the room, the building, the area of town, the whole city and beyond.

Doing this on a daily basis you will begin to feel very relaxed and ready to move on to the work at hand. All that happens is that your mind is allowed to escape for a few moments from the rush of normal activity. You are flexing neurological muscles not normally used.

Relaxation and meditation enable us to tap into unused resources. Experiencing the quiet within you gives you an added dimension – a still centre – from which to relate to yourself and your world. You become less blown about by events and other people, and more stable in your own understanding or perspective.

What About Sleep?

Deep, regenerative sleep is a primary requirement for good health. During deep sleep we allow stress, held in the muscles of the body, to release. It is the only time of the day when the immune system rebuilds.

The lack of sleep is cumulative; getting one good night's sleep does not make up for one bad night. The body needs good quality sleep for rejuvenation and repair. When we sleep our mind alternates between deeper and shallower levels of sleep. With each repetition of this cycle our body becomes more and more relaxed. Disruptions to this cycle mean we never get the full benefit of sleep.

It is a well-known fact that poor sleep is a major cause of automotive accidents and work accidents. It is also a contributor to alcoholism. Often a person with problems sleeping begins drinking before bed. Over time the need for alcohol increases until a dependency is established; the same situation occurs with drugs. Many who become dependent on drugs start out taking them to sleep.

In a study at the prestigious Henry Ford Hospital Sleep Disorders Centre, it was discovered that sleep is a major contributor to automobile accidents attributed to alcohol. In double-blind placebo studies it was found that incremental sleep deprivation vastly increased the subjects' tolerance for alcohol. Those who had a "sleep debt" were very prone to becoming very groggy with even a small amount of alcohol in their systems.

When we think about improving our well being, we usually only consider our diet and exercise. It really is amazing to think that sleep gets such little attention, especially as we feel so good when we have been sleeping well. Sleep is the basis of good health and the foundation of overall wellness. Sleep deprivation is one of the most effective means of torture. Scientific studies show that better quality sleep can enhance your life in many areas, such as your immune system, energy levels, concentration, physical restoration and the rate at which you learn things.

Many of us are not getting the recommended 7–8 hours of good, deep quality sleep each night. The reasons for this are varied, the main ones being stress, physical discomfort and inferior bedding/mattress quality. When assessing your sleeping patterns, it is important to look at a number of elements.

Don't Count Sheep – Count Your Blessings

We have talked quite a bit about stress and how to relieve it so far. Difficulty in sleeping is where stress takes its greatest toll. When the time comes to rest and sink into deep sleep, we can't. The stresses of the day start their re-runs, and the body is still armoured for attack. This is often when the Million Monkeys come out to play in earnest. Before going to bed is not the time to review everything that went wrong during the day.

What is on your mind when you go to sleep is what you sleep with. If you use some of the relaxation exercises listed above, they can help you get into a more relaxed frame of mind. A review of what is good is a good idea. Count your blessings. Some people might think that's a naive or loopy idea, but to me the alternative is what's weird. OK, I'm not always able to do it, but I always try that first, so most of the time I go to sleep thinking about the people I love and the things I love to do. Sometimes I do some affirmations. It really helps.

Take a look at your mattress – it's one household item that often gets neglected. How many times have you lain down on a bed and rolled into the deep pit in the middle?

A good mattress needs to provide firm support for the back, allowing the spine to stretch out in the night. If you are sleeping on a cream puff, it may feel cosy when you climb into bed but the question is, how does it help you sleep?

We all sweat at night. Most of us aren't aware of it, but we all lose about a cup of water when we sleep. Much of this perspiration soaks into the mattress. This, combined with the old skin that flakes off, provides a perfect medium for dust mites and mildew. This is especially true in a damp climate like the UK. This can increase irritation in the sinuses and lungs.

The effect of a bad mattress can be enormous. If moisture builds up between the skin surface and the bedding, the body will shift in order to dry the skin. If your mattress is too soft you will get into a twisted position and wake with stiff muscles. Make sure you air your bedding and flip your mattress regularly. You might even think about getting something revolutionary to sleep on.

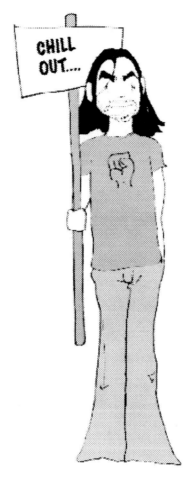

In the first chapter I told you about my experience with a magnetic mattress. Since that time I have met hundreds of people who had similar experiences. This is one of those things that is easy to dismiss as a placebo effect. Something isn't supposed to work, but it does, so what's really happening? I am a simple girl but isn't that what science is supposed to be the most interested in? What interests me is that in so many cases where something works that isn't supposed to, the critics don't even bother to do serious testing. Magnetic health products are a fine example.

I had an experience that was very positive. Sleeping on a magnetic sleep system seemed to relax my body to such a degree that some of my symptoms simply went away. I believe that when stress is released, the body is more capable of healing itself. Nothing else had worked and I must say I didn't expect this to either. After all . . . magnets?

After I had my experience I began to do some research and some thinking and it all made sense to me. Everything in the body operates on bioelectrical principles. Acupuncture and many other Asian health practices rely on stimulating or re-balancing this life energy. I referred to it earlier as "chi" or life force. One type of chi was called Earth Energy, that's close enough for me. Since we live on a big magnet (planet earth) and the magnetic field of the planet is essential for life, why wouldn't it be? We know that ancient people around the world used magnetic minerals for health care.

A wonderful thing is that there is increasing research being done on the applications of magnets for health. Several universities are engaged in a wide variety of clinical trials for the therapeutic application of magnetic fields for a range of health problems; medicine will come around sooner or later. Some studies have shown that blood circulation is increased with the application of weak magnetic fields. That's great because the energy is so safe; but you don't have to wait until then. Products are already there for you that can help you reduce stress and get a good night's sleep.

I learned that there was one company, Nikken, which had done its homework and produced safe products that were based on the most up-to-date research. They made the bed that was so helpful to me. One thing that I liked about them and their products was that they made no wild claims about healing anything. They created products that help you to relax and reduce stress. When I sleep on my magnetic mattress I wake up ready to go. So do all the clients I have introduced to this wonderful technology. In case you are wondering, they don't pay me to say this.

Finally, A Good Night's Sleep

Dear Marlene,

When I first met you I was having trouble sleeping. I would waken about 2a.m. and just couldn't get back to sleep. With my three children, Edward, Bethan and William to look after this left me feeling exhausted during the day.

I started your Chi Ball Classes and booked personal training sessions with you that involved power walking with my new cardio-strides. Both have increased my strength, stamina and energy levels.

When I purchased my magnetic sleep system, the

mattress and pillow were a little hard to get used to but you re-assured me and told me my body would eventually love it. You were right of course. I now sleep like a log and if I wake up I get back to sleep very easily. My husband Graham has also benefited from this wonderful concept.

You certainly are contagious Marlene as my Mother, Sister and Brother-in-law followed suit and absolutely love their magnetic pillows.

I now have my dog Nora and with my renewed energy have fun walking with her everyday. Thank you for everything.

Love

Gerry Campbell

Sleep Toolbox

Proper nutrition can help our sleep; dehydration can cause us to stay awake. Don't snack late at night or drink alcoholic beverages, tea or coffee for several hours before you sleep.

Apply some of the relaxation techniques listed in this earlier when in bed.

Try to reduce noise; don't fall asleep in front of the TV or with the radio on.

Don't watch disruptive programmes on TV or even the news late in the evening. Try reading instead.

Wear a comfortable eye mask to block out light.

Getting good exercise during the day will contribute to a better night's sleep.

Don't review the day's problems before sleep. This is a dedicated time for your body to rest; respect it.

CHAPTER NINE
A HEALTHY HABITAT

This is a short chapter but it is a very important one. When you mention the word environment people usually think about the world outside, they think of nature. I want to talk about two different environments: the one we live in, our homes, offices and schools, as well as the outside world. This is an important distinction because we are increasingly seeing nature as an alien place that we only sometimes visit. For most people the environment they live in is the built one, the indoor one.

Recent studies have shown that most people who live in cities are only outside 10% of the time. Just the short walk from the house to the car or from the door to the bus stop is the outdoor time. We are becoming creatures insulated from the outside world. Like in some science-fiction movie we are huddled up indoors, shut away from the world. Some of this insulation is good. I'm sure that the cave was draughty; who needs animals wandering in when you're trying to cook dinner?

All benefits of physical comfort aside, we have created some problems as well. Just as we need food that our bodies recognize to be healthy, we need exposure to nature for both body and mind. There are gifts in nature that are not only pleasant, but also essential for health. The simple reason for this is that nature is coded in our bodies and minds. The sights and sounds of nature, waves on the shore, the colour of a sunset, speak directly from the source of our being. Nature produces a state of calm because it is our source. For me, a person who is healthy is a person who respects nature and lives in a way that does the least damage to it.

When we are surrounded by the noise and sensorial overload of modern living, it is important to create an oasis of calm to relax and recharge in. If we take a little time and expend a little energy we can create a living space that gives up the stress-free zone we need. City living involves immersion in chaos, the natural environment is one of order. We need a sense of order around us so that we can shake off chaos and stress just as we need the nourishment of sunshine, clean air and clean water to live.

The Stress-free Zone

In the past few years the ancient Chinese art of Feng Shui has become popular. Home magazines regularly feature houses that have been arranged using the principles of the art. Usually they are spacious places with sparse furnishing. They sometimes don't look like anyone lives there at all, or at least anyone with children or pets. The aim is to produce a living space that is peaceful and stress free. I am not a feng shui practitioner but I know that your house can either stress you out or have a calming effect. My sisters and I have always had a knack for creating peaceful homes. When others come in they always comment on how calming it is to be there. Here are some of the things I think are important.

Everyone has his or her own sense of comfortable surroundings, but clutter is clutter. In de-stressing your home, get the clutter under control first. Instead of loading every shelf in a room with books and mementos, store some away and cycle them back in a few months. Here is a news flash – it is even possible to throw things away. Recycle what you don't need or take them to an Oxfam shop so someone else can use them.

When there is clutter around you, it serves as a distraction that you become used to. It takes up space in your mind that needs clearing. Look at your house and imagine that you are looking at your brain. What does it say about your thought processes? This is an easy task. Take a day just to de-clutter your house. Tidy your drawers and clean off your surfaces. You will feel better for it.

Look at the way that your rooms are furnished. It can make a huge difference if you can navigate your rooms easily. Sometimes we may place chairs or sofas so that they protrude into the natural movement of people through the room; remove the roadblocks. If you have a piece of furniture you always bump into, move it or remove it.

Light is important. This may seem superficial, but the amount of light in your home can make the difference between feeling happy or depressed. Having a house that looks like a nightclub may be fine on Saturday night, but what about the rest of the week? Clean windows and light colours are helpful as a backdrop for relaxation and lightness of spirit. These are little things that can make the difference.

A sense of order doesn't need to be set aside because there are children in the house. I know many people who have managed to create relaxing homes with children. It is worth setting up rewards for keeping rooms tidy and especially those rooms that are used by the whole family. Giving children assignments to help keep the home clean can give them a sense of being responsible.

Every Breath You Take

Recent studies have shown what many of us have known since we were children: nature has a therapeutic effect. Our nervous system responds differently to the sounds and rhythms of nature than it does to the noise of a city street. When we walk in the woods or beach or alongside a running stream, our senses are not only being soothed, we also benefit greatly by exposure to negative ions in the air. These "air vitamins" stimulate a feeling of well being and happiness.

There is a high concentration of negative ions in nature. Areas where there is running water, waterfalls, dense plant life and at the seashore all have very high concentrations. In these locations it is easy to feel positive. The opposite is true with positive ions; these are found in areas where the traffic is concentrated or there is a high concentration of machines or computer terminals. Positive ions make us feel irritable. I know that it's confusing that it's the negative ones that make us positive, but that's the wonderful world of science.

Unless the air outside is really bad, filled with traffic fumes, giving your house an airing regularly is a very good idea. Even in the winter, just opening the windows for about 10 minutes can make a difference for the rest of the day. Keeping healthy plants in your house can increase negative ions in your home, but make sure that you keep them healthy. A dead plant is . . . well, dead.

Modern homes are often very well sealed in order to reduce fuel bills. The savings are a good idea but often keeping the air in isn't. The Environmental Protection Agency in America found that in many cities, the indoor air was more polluted than the air outside. The reason for this has to do with the fact that many toxic materials are used in creating modern furnishings. Adhesives used in furniture (especially inexpensive furniture) and to keep carpets or flooring in place are highly toxic and continue to out-gas for months and even years. This is in addition to the use of toxic substances for cleaning, often kept in the house with lids not properly sealed. These chemical gases combined with bacteria, viruses and dust, can create a potent cocktail for someone with respiratory challenges, let alone someone with healthy lungs.

If negative ions can be introduced into a home or office environment, it is a huge benefit to the health of everyone who breathes it. The negative ions leach the positive ions out of the air as well as reducing the amount of dust particles in the air. This is true since most dust particles are positively charged. The same phenomenon also seems to be the case in dealing with many microbes. Studies in America and the UK have shown that the introduction of ions was effective in reducing the bacterial and viral content of the air. There are products on the market that can filter the air and products that introduce negative ions, but having both is ideal.

In the last chapter I talked about the magnetic mattress that was so instrumental in my recovery from my back injury. The same company, Nikken, makes two other products that I feel are essential to my healthy home. The Pi Water system and the Air Power 5 are technologies that

I consider superior to anything else on the market. They work and I am happy to recommend them. If you can find anything better, let me know.

The Air Power 5 System

The Nikken air system provides several benefits. To clean the air the system uses a HEPA filter in which a series of traps filter out both small and large particles from the air. HEPA (high efficiency particulate air) filters are the type used in operating theatres and in "clean rooms" in the electronics industry. The air then passes through to a photo catalytic filter that destroys pollutants and micro-organisms and a carbon filter that absorbs contaminants. You see why I am impressed - but there is more. In addition to filtering the air, the Air Power 5 does more. It produces those negative ions that I was talking about above and adds them back into the clean air. This is why I feel so much more alert when I am working on my computer for long hours and why I notice the difference of the air in my kitchen when I am cooking.

The Air Power 5 unit does all this without production of ozone, using a unique system that uses available light. Some companies produce ionization machines but they make the ions using technologies that discharge ozone as a by-product. Ozone is a contaminant, so cleaning the air and polluting it at the same time seems strange. So I get my ions straight, no ozone, thank you. After my magnetic mattress, my Air Power 5 is the third thing I would pack in the truck if I moved house. The second thing I would take would be my water system.

Water – The Key to Life

Everyone who knows me knows I am a water fanatic. When I talk to people about how bad the water that comes out of the tap is, they often get very defensive. It's almost as if bad water would be the last straw. We don't want to know. This is probably because we all feel deep down that water should be clean and free, and it should. It becomes a matter of civic pride. We know that there is something ridiculous about buying water in plastic bottles at a high price; what's next – private air? Let me tell you that when I changed my attitude about water and began using water that was not only pure but also processed for maximum health, I noticed the difference within weeks. My skin felt softer, my digestion improved and I felt more vigorous than ever before. My clients notice the same thing.

All biological life depends on water. It is the most important nutrient we consume. It is what we are made of. The human body is about 75% water. Our brain is 85% water. Take away the water and we are just a small pile of minerals. We know the importance and yet the monkeys all come out to play when the topic comes up.

Let's start with your garden. You all know that fertilizer makes your lawn turn green; it makes it healthier and more resistant to pests and disease. It makes the grass grow more quickly and appear more vibrant and healthy. That's the food part; fertilizer (natural, you know) is a basic nutrition for your lawn. I have yet to hear someone say there is no link between fertilizer and healthy lawns. The same is true with water. When there is a dry spell and you don't water your lawn, it turns brown and dies. We don't wet the lawn down with fizzy drinks or beer or coffee. The requirement is for water not liquid. We need water in the purest natural state possible for good health.

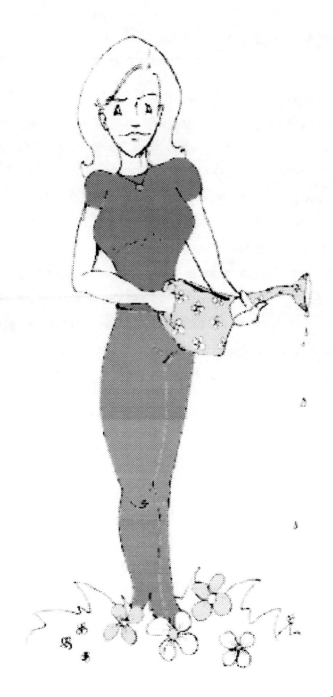

We all know that there has been deception in the bottled water industry. All you have to do is put something natural-looking on the label, like a tree or a mountain, remove the chlorine from some tap water and you're in business. Not all companies do that but some have succeeded in this con game. That shouldn't put us off looking seriously at the issue. The quality of water that we drink is very important to our health.

When we think of where we get our water, we usually think of deep aquifers where the water has trickled down through hundreds of feet of soil, been stripped of toxins and then percolated back up. What a fantasy. The water we drink has usually been pumped from a river that is contaminated with farm run-off and industrial waste. It is filtered just enough to pass the regulations, pumped up with a mega dose of chemicals to kill off all the bacterial matter and then drained off into large holding tanks where it sits, stagnant, until it is pumped through a decaying system of pipes till it emerges from your tap. Wow, did I just write that sentence? Is it any wonder that the consumption of bottled water is rising so fast or that people drink so many other beverages instead of tap water?

Our ability to absorb water decreases with age, due to the amount of toxins we ingest over time in our food and drink. As these toxins build up, cells are unable to absorb water effectively and eliminate toxins. While a newborn baby may be 90% hydrated, a person of 65 years, for instance, will be about 50% hydrated. Most of the difference is cellular hydration. The British Dietetic Association advises that adults consume 2.5 litres of water daily. This means water, not liquid.

This dehydration has several causes: junk foods, foods which have been treated with chemicals or pesticides, the wrong balance of food, eating foods out of season, air pollution, travelling in aircraft, air conditioning, drinking coffee and fizzy drinks, just to name a few. The body needs water to flush toxins that are a natural product of metabolism as well as those we take in. Some of our habits confuse the body. We drink alcohol, coffee or fizzy drinks and the body wants to get rid of the toxins or becomes dehydrated by caffeine and sends a message of thirst so we drink more of the same. What's a body to do?

This may be one of the reasons why the sizes of drinks are getting bigger and bigger. In America the drinks in restaurants and movie theatres look like buckets and the trend is growing here. We want to hydrate but aren't able to satisfy the deep biological need with what we are drinking. We want a large drink with ice – this complicates the problem.

The body gets very confused when it tries to make a balance and can't get what it needs. By eating a diet that produces an acid condition in the stomach, we not only crave water, we also crave something to cool down the acid stomach. It is more and more common for people to want their drinks chilled, especially water. Notice how ice in water has become common. We are trying to settle down a violently disturbed stomach. When we drink chilled drinks, the stomach spasms. It takes some time but if you are eating a good diet you will find that drinking water at room temperature is much more satisfying.

By drinking the best water possible, our cells will absorb it more easily and readily and will stop us from feeling the effects of everyday dehydration: headaches, a lack of concentration, constipation, dry skin and increased stress levels. There are many who believe that the poor quality of our water is a contributing factor to many degenerative diseases, allergies, hypertension, obesity and emotional problems such as depression. Let's take a look at just one aspect of illness: arteriosclerosis. Before the turn of the century arteriosclerosis was unknown.

Arteriosclerosis is a hardening of the arteries characterized by the gradual accumulation of fatty substances embedded in the inner wall of the blood vessels, making the passage of blood more difficult and putting a greater workload on the heart. The medical profession would have us think that the problem is primarily dietary. Diet is only part of the problem. People have been eating fatty foods for centuries.

An American physician, Dr Price, investigated an interesting fact in his 1969 publication, *Coronary/Cholesterol/Chlorine*. He noted a high rate of arteriosclerosis among servicemen in Vietnam. Under combat conditions there was no room for gastrointestinal disorders, so chlorine concentrations in the drinking water were maintained at a very high level. He noticed unusually high rates of cholesterol in 18 and 20-year-old men, and eventually arrived at the conclusion that this was caused by chlorinated water. He went on to prove his theory under controlled conditions with chickens, some given chlorinated water and others a diet without chlorine. The theory was borne out, but unless you have happened to come across this little known publication, you have never heard of Dr Price or his discovery. Since all tap water is treated with chlorine we should be interested in this.

Listen to what Dr Bercz of the Cincinnati Laboratory has to say. "Studies in non-human primates have shown that the chlorine treated water causes depression of high density lipoprotein (HDL) bound cholesterol, shifting the binding to the low density form (LDL). The protection of the former and the role of the LDL in coronary heart disease is an established medical fact." We need to pay attention because this is a health issue that is easy to ignore. We get used to bad water and soon we can't tell the difference any more or we simply stop drinking it.

If you are using an effective filtration system, you are ahead of the game. It is important to get the rubbish out, including as much of the chlorine as possible. Carbon filters are effective depending on the design and the type of carbon used and there are many on the market. There are also reverse osmosis filters, but they are not as efficient.

Ever since I became interested in alternative health, the issue of pure water has drawn my attention. After being introduced to the magnetic products of Nikken I discovered another product they were distributing that really impressed me when I started using it. It was called the Nikken Pi Water System. What makes it unique is that it goes beyond simply filtering out the toxins, it attempts to restore the water to its natural state.

Pi Water

I know people who heard about this Pi system twenty years ago. It was invented in Japan and was very expensive. About five years ago I was at a convention in Australia where this system was being launched. I was nearly out of my seat with excitement (sad perhaps) but none the less I was over the moon to be able to order my own. They are now available in the UK. The unit is free standing and easy to assemble. I use it for everything, from drinking pi water, making tea, soups, cooking grains and even use it as a "spritzer" on my face. It is fantastic for hydrating your skin when you are indoors with central heating. I use it on my plants and they have never looked healthier.

The Japanese researchers who created the system were trying to replicate the water in a specific river that supported very abundant plant growth. They studied the water and discovered that when they mimicked the characteristics of the water, plants and other organisms flourished. Nikken improved on the technology and introduced it in the West.

The Pi system uses mined coral, block charcoal, charcoal fragments, ceramics, natural anti-fungal minerals and magnetic energy to produce clean "living water" from ordinary tap water. Aside from filtering the water to a very high standard, the exposure to the special ceramic beads in the unit allows trace minerals and calcium ions to leach into the water. This process helps the body to reduce acidity and establish a healthy Ph factor. The use of magnets to "energize" the water makes it easier to absorb into the body.

When I started using the water I noticed several differences in my health. Firstly there was a change in my skin. I have always had good skin but I could feel it becoming softer. This made sense to me because hydration can affect the collagen matrix that breaks down and decreases with age, causing wrinkles. Oh my, exciting news.

I also noticed that my digestion improved. Since having my gall bladder removed, I had some problems and the water seemed to make things much better. Since then I have had many clients who have reported that they noticed similar effects. The most exciting thing, though, was that I started drinking more water, I craved it.

When my clients started drinking Pi water they noticed that their cravings for other drinks diminished. What great news. Some noticed that their children were interested in drinking water, which came as a shock.

Nikken has now come out with a new technology, which has given the whole water issue a new dimension. The Optimiser spins the pure water, creating a vortex that aerates it in a magnetic field, adding more oxygen. I make beautiful water at home for pennies and take it with me when I am out, or use the portable filter bottle that they make. I never buy bottled water but I always have the best water available.

Occasional Unplugging

Particularly if we live in a city, we are continually surrounded by uninvited information – television, radios, street noise and the usual background sounds. One habit that is very common is to invite more tension into the house when we get home. I know that some people get a great deal of pleasure from watching a good movie or a sporting event on TV. There are programmes that are funny, informative or entertaining; I also know that it can dominate a whole house. To alleviate stress and allow the body and mind to relax, try unplugging. To much TV often serves to deflect our attention from our own lives. Just see what it's like to wean off the tube if you are stuck in front of it every night.

Reading, listening to music, picking up an old hobby or just experiencing the quiet can all add a new dimension. If you have a big family and there is lots of activity, wait until the kids go to bed or organize games or activities that don't require the TV. It's worth a try.

Something For The Whole Family

Dear Marlene,

What a wonderful time we had at our family consultation with you last Sunday at your Studio. My husband Alistair and I were thrilled at how much our kids enjoyed the experience. Emma, Jenna, Katie and Laura are now enjoying sprouting their own seeds, making delicious smoothies and planning menus for us all. You have definitely made a huge difference to what they eat and Laura aged four keeps asking, "Would Marlene let me eat this Mum". Emma and Jenna are moving towards being vegetarian and found your information invaluable and were delighted with the recipes that you gave us.

Ever since I bought the Pi Water System, the kids drink lots of water and less juice and even Ben our dog loves the Pi Water.

They all loved your Chi Ball Class and wish this could be part of their PE at school.

We all want to say a huge thank you Marlene for making life easier by simplifying nutrition, giving us some great ideas and steering us all towards a much healthier lifestyle.

Janice Clyne
The Sano Spa

Healthy Home Toolbox

De-clutter – if you don't use things, get rid of them. If there is too much stuff store it.

Let there be light – clean the windows. Light is so important. Think about having the most light and brightness in your home and it will ease your mind.

Clear the space. If there is anything you bump into get rid of it or move it. There is no need to have your subconscious mind worrying about the next bang on the shin.

Breathe easy – aromatherapy. Aroma therapy is the use of smells to calm the mind. Smell is a powerful trigger to the emotions. Different smells can make us feel calm, alert, sexy or sleepy. Experiment with candles or aroma therapy oils and find out which sents help you establish the aroma zone that you like best.

(The Air Power 5 unit has an aroma therapy attachment).

Keep the kitchen clean. If you are eating a healthy diet and cooking more of your own food it is important to keep the kitchen inviting and ready to go. If you come home from work and the kitchen is messy, with dishes in the sink you will be more likely to avoid cooking a good meal. You can check this out with yourself. If the kitchen is clean and everything is put away you will be more inspired to be creative in the kitchen.

The Last Word

I really do hope that my little book has been helpful to you. I know that if you pick up even some of the ideas I have talked about and incorporate them into your life you will be better for it. We all deserve to live our life to the fullest, to have all the health and vitality possible so that we can pursue our personal dreams. Health is about forming habits that serve our personal purpose. If I have helped you do that then I have moved one step closer to fulfilling my purpose - to help in the creation of a healthy world. I want to leave you with my favourite quote from a farmer in the American South called Eubie Blake who was

100 years old when he said, "If I had known I was going to live this long, I would have taken better care of myself." God Bless.

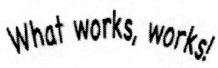

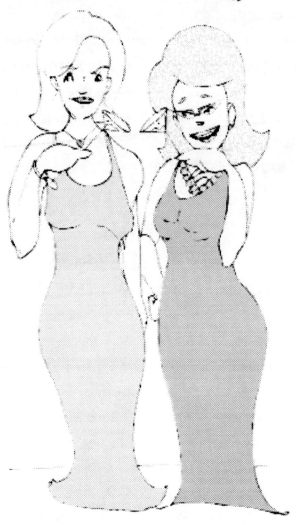

CHAPTER TEN
THE NO NONSENSE HEALTH QUIZ AND WORKSHEETS

Personal Health Assessment

The purpose of this questionnaire is to help you determine which Body Design Balance Lifestyle Programme path will best suit you. Please answer the questionnaire completely by choosing only one from each question. Once you've done this, total your points.

How would you describe your physical appearance?

Fit and lean   1 point _____

Average   2 points_____

Slightly overweight   3 points_____

Overweight   4 points_____

How often do you currently work out?

5 + times a week   1 point _____

3–4 times a week   2 points_____

1–2 times a week   3 points_____

1–2 times a month   4 points_____

Never   5 points_____

What is your exercise intensity level?

High	1 point	_____
Moderate	2 points	_____
Low	3 points	_____

How do you currently eat?

Smaller meals and snacks throughout the day	1 point	_____
Three meals a day	2 points	_____
Skip meals	3 points	_____
Eat more than 3 regular-sized meals daily	4 points	_____

Which of the following best describes your current eating habits?

Eat healthy	1 point	_____
Skip meals	2 points	_____
Continuous snacker	3 points	_____
Junk food junkie	4 points	_____

What do your meals consist of?

5 portions of fruit and vegetables

daily or more	1 point	_____
Fairly healthy – not consistent	2 points	_____
Conventional diet	3 points	_____
Fast food/packaged meals	4 points	_____

How often do you have chocolate, sweet desserts or fizzy drinks daily?

0–1 times per day	1 point	_____
1–2 times per day	2 points	_____
2–4 times a day	3 points	_____
5 + times a day	4 points	_____

How many glasses of water a day do you drink?

6–8 glasses	1 point	_____
4–6 glasses	2 points	_____
2–4 glasses	3 points	_____
1–2 glasses	4 points	_____

How much time are you willing to put into a fitness programme?

3 + hours/week   1 point _____

1.5–3 hours/week   2 points_____

0–1.5 hours/week   3 points_____

Do you take a nutritional supplement?

Everyday   1 point _____

Sometimes   2 points_____

Never   3 points_____

Do you smoke?

Never   1 point _____

On occasion   3 points_____

Daily   5 points_____

How many units of alcohol do you consume weekly?
Female

0–5   1 point _____

5–7   2 points_____

Over 7   3 points_____

Male

0–5	1 point _____
7–10	2 points_____
Over 14	3 points_____

Total Points ....

17 POINTS OR LESS

If your total is 17 or below you are looking after your well being and simply need to continue with health maintenance.

17–23 POINTS

You need to make some adjustments to increase fitness levels and to improve your prevention score. Pick key areas that you are not now working on and improve them.

23–29 POINTS

You need a structured and disciplined programme to improve your general fitness.

OVER 29 POINTS

It is important that you make a firm commitment to improving your health with a focused exercise and dietary programme. Act now so that you can enjoy a healthy life.

Your Food Journal

As you change your diet, you may find that keeping a food journal is a good idea. Many of my clients have found it very helpful. The journal will help you keep track of what you really eat and often why you eat it. Your journals can also be used to track patterns of eating that you would never have noticed.

Since your body is always trying to make balance, you may see that a particular work habit, family situation or activity influences what you eat the next day. It is fascinating to see the patterns that can emerge. Just copy this form out on a piece of paper and make copies.

The goal at first is simply to make a record of what you eat without any judgement. The first week should be interesting. Now go back and read the chapters on food again.

Daily Food
Today's Portions   This Week

Wholegrain
Refined Grain or Commercial Bread
Vegetables (cooked)
Vegetables (raw)
Beans or Vegetable Protein
Fish

Fruit

Nuts or Seeds

Sea Vegetables

Jade GreenZymes

Green Tea

Herbal Tea

Coffee

Black Tea

Fruit Juice

Fizzy Drinks

Fish

Eggs

Fowl

Red Meat

Milk

Cheese

Yoghurt

Pudding

Sweets

Sugared Baked Goods

Wine

Beer

Spirits

Your Fitness Journal

This really is a great journal to use. My clients tell me that even looking at their journal lying on the coffee table is enough to make them squirm if it's not been opened for a few days so they go out for a quick 30 minute power walk to get back on track. Be it the gym, walking, cycling or whatever, fill in whatever activities you have been doing and log the time. Set new goals to increase the duration.

Daily Goal …….. Time ……..
Type of Exercise ……..

Weekly Goal …….. Time ……..
Type of Exercise………

Monthly Goal …….. Time ……..
Type of Exercise………

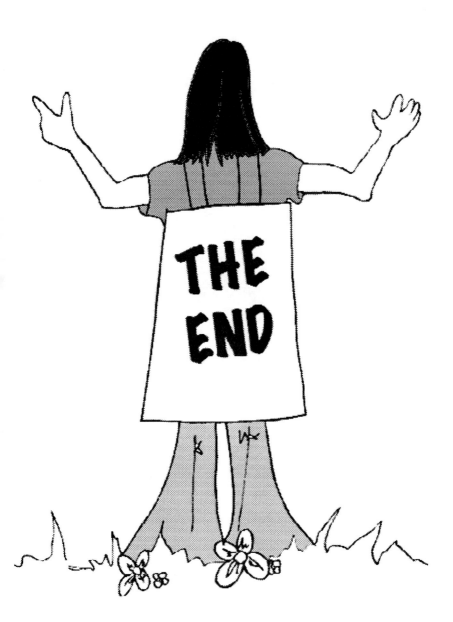